THE TOP 100
FITNESS
FOODS

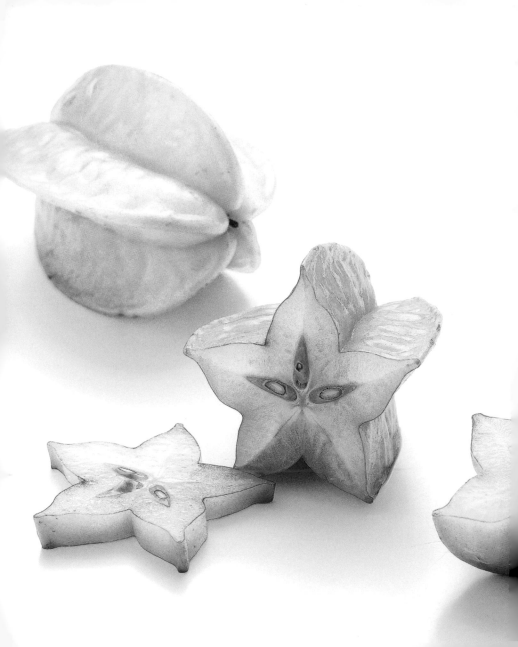

THE TOP 100 FITNESS FOODS

SARAH OWEN

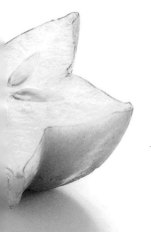

DUNCAN BAIRD PUBLISHERS

LONDON

THE TOP 100 FITNESS FOODS
Sarah Owen

First published in the United Kingdom and Ireland in 2009 by
Duncan Baird Publishers Ltd
Sixth Floor, Castle House
75–76 Wells Street
London W1T 3QH

Conceived, created and designed by Duncan Baird Publishers

Managing Editors: Grace Cheetham and Deirdre Headon
Editor: Ingrid Court-Jones
Managing Designer: Suzanne Tuhrim
Designer: Jantje Doughty
Commissioned photography: Simon Smith and Toby Scott

British Library Cataloguing-in-Publication Data:
A CIP record for this book is available from the British Library

ISBN: 978-1-84483-869-1

10 9 8 7 6 5 4 3 2 1

Typeset in Helvetica Condensed
Colour reproduction by Colourscan, Singapore
Printed in Malaysia by Imago

Publisher's Note: The information in this book is not intended as a substitute for professional
medical advice and treatment. If you are pregnant or breastfeeding or have any special dietary
requirements, allergies or medical conditions, it is recommended that you consult a medical
professional before following any of the information or recipes contained in this book. Duncan
Baird Publishers, or any other persons who have been involved in working on this publication,
cannot accept responsibility for any errors or omissions, inadvertent or not, that may be found
in the recipes or text, nor for any problems that may arise as a result of preparing one of these
recipes or following the advice contained in this work.

Notes on the recipes
Unless otherwise stated:
• All recipes serve 4 • Use fresh herbs • Do not mix metric and Imperial measurements
• 1 tsp = 5ml, 1 tbsp = 15ml, 1 cup = 250ml • All fruit, vegetables and eggs are medium-sized
unless specified otherwise.

CONTENTS

KEY TO SYMBOLS

 energy-boosting

 rehydrating

 joint-friendly

 bone-strengthening

 muscle-building

 stamina-improving

 blood sugar-balancing

 cramp-preventing

introduction

With soaring rates of obesity in the West, more people than ever before are taking responsibility for their own health and following a fitness regime or taking up a sport. Regardless of whether they're an absolute beginner or a world-class professional, all athletes have one thing in common – unique nutritional demands, which require them to top up their energy tank with enough fuel to keep them going until the end of a match, a race, an aerobics class or a gym session.

It's been proven time and time again that diet can have a significant impact on everything from speed and stamina to post-workout recovery rates. Here's what's needed to guarantee peak performance every time.

CARBOHYDRATE
Converted into glycogen, carbohydrates are the body's main source of energy and are stored in the muscles, where they're used as fuel during activity. Research shows that regular exercisers need to consume approximately 50–60 per cent of their total calorie intake in carbohydrates to maximize their performance.

One of the healthiest and most convenient sources of readily absorbed carbohydrates is fruit, which provides a quick energy boost as well as helping to rehydrate the body. Unrefined grains, such as oats and brown rice, are rich in slow-releasing carbohydrates, which help to feed the muscles steadily and sustain them for endurance events.

EAT TO STAY FIT

STAY HYDRATED

Of all the nutrients, water is the most important. It makes up more than 60 per cent of body weight and is vital for the functioning of all cells. You need to top up your fluid levels regularly because water is lost through sweating, breathing and urine, sapping endurance and strength. Even mild dehydration can result in fatigue, as the body is unable to cool itself efficiently, and losing the equivalent of 2 per cent of body weight in sweat results in a 10–20 per cent drop in aerobic capacity. Experts recommend drinking six to eight glasses of water a day, and possibly more in hot weather and during particularly intense bouts of exercise.

BEFORE EXERCISE

Research has found that it's best to eat a light carbohydrate-based meal or snack two to four hours before exercise. This should leave enough time for the body to partially digest the food so that you don't feel nauseous. The resulting rise in blood-glucose levels allows the body to exercise harder and longer. Some studies also show that eating three hours before exercise helps the body to burn more fat. It's best not to eat a big meal just before working out, though, as that's likely to lead to performance-impairing sluggishness.

DURING EXERCISE

Anyone exercising for longer than 30 minutes benefits from sipping water periodically, while if a workout lasts longer than 60 minutes, studies have shown that eating a high-carbohydrate snack can top up blood-sugar levels to help the body to keep going for longer. Fast-burning carbohydrates, such as a banana or a cereal bar, work particularly well. Isotonic drinks are also a good option – these carbohydrate-rich drinks provide fuel for the muscles and help to speed up the absorption of water into the bloodstream.

AFTER EXERCISE

Whether or not you feel hungry, the quicker you consume food or drink after a workout, the quicker your body will recover. The enzymes that make glycogen (muscle fuel) are most active between 30 minutes and two hours after exercise. In fact, carbohydrate is converted into glycogen one-and-a-half times faster than normal during this post-exercise window. Wait more than two hours and the body's ability to reload muscle glycogen drops by 66 per cent. Including a little protein in a snack speeds up glycogen recovery even further. Research shows that the perfect post-exercise meal or snack is made up of three parts carbohydrate to one part protein – this ratio boosts glycogen storage by almost 40 per cent.

USEFUL INFORMATION

• Each recipe serves four unless otherwise specified.

• Feel free to adjust the quantities and ingredients in the recipes to suit individual tastes.

• Wash all fruit and vegetables thoroughly unless they're organic, in which case a quick rinse under the tap will do.

• Beans, especially kidney beans, can be poisonous if not cooked properly. Tinned beans are a safe, nutritious alternative. If using dried beans, soak them for least five hours. Throw away the water and boil them in two to three times their volume of water fresh water for 10 minutes, then cook them for at least one hour. Avoid slow cookers, which don't reach a high enough temperature to cook them thoroughly – undercooked beans are more poisonous than raw ones.

• Green and brown lentils need to be soaked; red lentils don't.

• Always clean seafood thoroughly, discarding any with shells that are broken or already open. Don't eat any whose shells remain closed when cooked.

• Meat should be cooked through. Don't burn it, though, as this can create chemical reactions that have been linked with cancer.

PROTEIN

Protein is vital for the growth, formation and repair of body cells and for making enzymes, hormones and antibodies. It is also important for bone health.

Anyone who's physically active needs to eat more protein to make up for the increased muscle breakdown that occurs during and after exercise. The amount depends on the type of sport and intensity of the workout. Endurance athletes, such as long-distance runners, need between 1.2 and 1.4g (0.04–0.05oz) of protein per kilogram (2lb 4oz) of body weight; anyone who concentrates on strength activities, such as weight training, needs between 1.4 and 1.8g (0.05–0.06oz) per kilogram (2lb 4oz) of body weight a day. This is approximately 20–25 per cent of overall calorie intake. Excellent sources of protein include lean meat and poultry, fish, dairy products, pulses, soya, nuts and seeds.

FAT

A concentrated source of energy, fat also provides the body with some important nutrients, such as vitamins A, D and E. It's recommended that anyone who works out or plays sport regularly should consume

20–25 per cent of their total daily calorie intake in fat. However, it's worth remembering that there are different types of fats, some of which are healthier for us than others. The so-called "bad", saturated fats (found in meat and dairy products) and hydrogenated fats (found in margarine, pastries, biscuits and fried food) have been linked to an increased risk of heart disease and stroke. Consequently, these should make up no more than 10 per cent of the total calories we consume in a day. The remaining 10–15 per cent of our calorie intake from fats should be made up of "good" fats – the monounsaturated fats (found in olives, avocados and peanuts) and the omega-3, -6 and -9 essential fatty acids (found in fish, nuts and seeds). These offer many benefits for athletes, including helping to reduce blood pressure and cholesterol levels, and working as an anti-inflammatory to protect joints.

VITAMINS AND MINERALS

Your body needs vitamins and minerals in minute amounts to help it to function at its best, and there's no doubt that getting the balance right boosts overall sports performance. Fresh fruit and vegetables are the richest sources of these important nutrients. Many vitamins, such as A, C and E, are also antioxidants, which counterbalance the potentially damaging effects of free radicals produced naturally during exercise. It's recommended that anyone who works out or plays sports regularly consumes five to seven portions of fruit and vegetables a day.

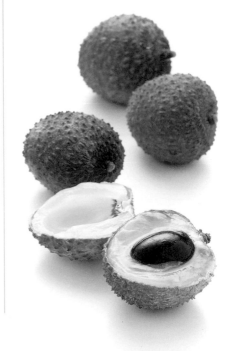

pear

NUTRIENTS

Vitamin C, beta-carotene, folic acid; calcium, iron, magnesium, phosphorus, potassium, zinc

Bursting with natural sugar that converts easily into energy, a pear is an ideal pre-workout snack.

One pear contains approximately one-tenth of the recommended daily intake of potassium, a mineral easily lost through perspiration. This is important for anyone who exercises because a lack of potassium can lead to fatigue and muscle cramps. Pears are also among the few fruits that contain lots of insoluble fibre, which works like tiny scrubbing brushes in the colon to promote good digestion.

POACHED PEARS

4 pears, peeled
100g/3½oz clear honey
125ml/4½fl oz/½ cup
    apple juice
1 tsp ground ginger

Place the pears in a pan and pour over the honey, juice and 250ml/9fl oz/1 cup water. Sprinkle over the ginger and bring to the boil. Reduce the heat, cover and simmer for 20 minutes. Allow to cool in the syrup.

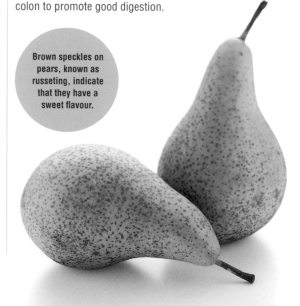

Brown speckles on pears, known as russeting, indicate that they have a sweet flavour.

banana

The ultimate fast food, bananas provide a potent mix of vitamins, minerals and carbohydrates.

Ripe bananas contain the ideal carbohydrate combination to replace muscle glycogen before or during exercise. Glucose, the most easily digested sugar, is immediately absorbed into the bloodstream for instant energy, while fructose is absorbed more slowly, providing a steady supply of fuel over a time. Bananas are also an excellent source of potassium and vitamin B6, which is involved in the manufacture of red blood cells as well as the breakdown of proteins, carbohydrates and fats.

NUTRIENTS
Vitamins B3, B5, B6, C, K, beta-carotene, folic acid; calcium, iron, magnesium, phosphorus, potassium, zinc

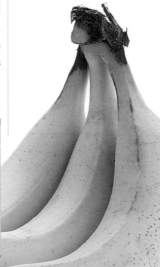

BREAKFAST SMOOTHIE *serves 2*

2 ripe bananas, peeled
20 raspberries
20 blueberries
500ml/17fl oz/2 cups
   natural bio-yogurt
½ tsp ground ginger

Whizz together the bananas, berries and yogurt in a blender until smooth. Pour into 2 glasses, sprinkle over the ginger and serve immediately.

plum

NUTRIENTS
Vitamins B2, C, beta-carotene; copper, potassium

This versatile fruit can be eaten fresh or dried and is a useful source of immunity-boosting antioxidants.

Plums are rich in pectin, a type of soluble fibre that absorbs and neutralizes toxins in the large intestine, which means that they have excellent detoxifying properties. They're great for helping to improve fitness in anaemia-prone athletes because they're packed with iron, which is crucial in the formation of red blood cells. They also contain malic acid and the antioxidant vitamin C, both of which enhance the absorption of iron.

PLUM COMPÔTE

16 ripe but firm plums
2 tsp ground allspice
2 tbsp dark brown sugar
250ml/9fl oz/1 cup
    orange juice
zest of ½ orange
natural bio-yogurt, to serve

Place the plums in a large ovenproof dish. Add the allspice, sugar, orange juice and zest, and bake in a pre-heated oven at 180°C/350°F/Gas mark 4 for 30 minutes. Serve with natural bio-yogurt.

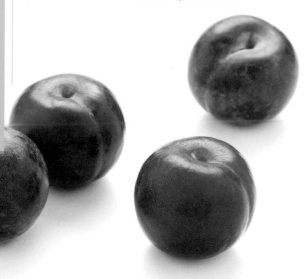

004

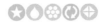

peach

This deliciously sweet treat helps to prevent dehydration – a common cause of fatigue.

A 2-per-cent loss of fluid can cause a 20-per-cent drop in energy, which is why dehydration is one of the major causes of fatigue during prolonged exercise. As well as drinking plenty of water, eating foods with a high water content, such as a ripe, juicy peach, is a good way to top up fluids. Peaches also contain the trace mineral boron, which affects the way the body metabolizes calcium and so is important for healthy bones.

NUTRIENTS
Vitamins B3, C, beta-carotene, folic acid; calcium, iron, magnesium, phosphorus, potassium, zinc

PEACHY FROZEN YOGURT

4 peaches, peeled
  and pitted
10 raspberries
10 strawberries, hulled
300ml/10½fl oz/1¼ cups
  natural bio-yogurt
juice of ½ lemon

Purée the fruit in a blender and place in a bowl in the freezer for 2–3 hours until semi-frozen. Remove and whisk in the yogurt and lemon juice. Freeze again until firm. Remove from the freezer 30 minutes before serving.

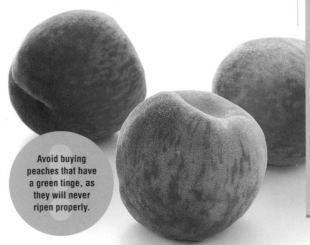

Avoid buying peaches that have a green tinge, as they will never ripen properly.

lemon

NUTRIENTS
Vitamins B3, B5, B6, C, E, beta-carotene, folic acid; calcium, copper, iodine, iron, magnesium, manganese, phosphorus, potassium, selenium, zinc

Bursting with antioxidants, lemons make a great addition to any fitness diet, whether as a flavouring in cooked dishes or simply squeezed over a salad.

Citric acid, which encourages healthy digestion, makes up 7 to 8 per cent of a lemon, the highest concentration found in any fruit. Try diluting freshly squeezed lemon juice with warm water and drinking it on an empty stomach first thing in the morning. Lemon juice is also one of the most concentrated food sources of vitamin C, making it the ideal addition to a glass of water to help soothe a post-exercise dry throat.

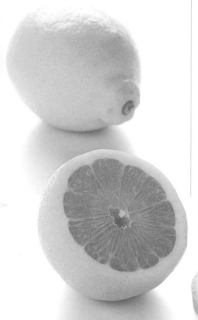

LEMONY STUFFING BALLS *makes 10*

1 small onion, quartered
1 egg, beaten
1 tbsp chopped rosemary
125g/4½oz/1½ cups fresh
white breadcrumbs
juice and zest of 1 lemon

Whizz the onion, egg and rosemary in a blender until smooth. In a bowl, mix the breadcrumbs with the lemon juice and zest, then combine the mixtures together. Form into 10 small balls. Place on a baking tray and bake in a pre-heated oven at 180°C/350°F/ Gas mark 4 for 25 minutes. Serve as an accompaniment.

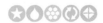

orange

The world's most popular citrus fruit is packed with infection-fighting and fat-burning nutrients.

Oranges contain natural sugars to help boost flagging energy levels and are full of vitamin C, a high intake of which can help to reduce post-exercise muscle soreness. They also provide citric acid, helping the body to absorb calcium, which is then stored in our fat cells. Oranges are a good source of the antioxidant hesperidin, thought to protect the heart by lowering cholesterol.

NUTRIENTS
Vitamins B3, B5, C, E, K, beta-carotene, folic acid; calcium, iodine, iron, magnesium, phosphorus, potassium, selenium, zinc

The bigger the "navel" in an orange, the sweeter it will be.

CHOCOLATE ORANGES

100g/3½oz plain chocolate, grated
1 tbsp golden syrup
zest of 1 orange
4 tbsp single cream
4 oranges, peeled

Put the grated chocolate and syrup in a heatproof bowl and gently melt over a pan of simmering water. Once they have melted, turn off the heat and stir in the zest and cream. Divide the oranges into segments and arrange on plates. Drizzle over the sauce and serve.

007

⭐🌀🌀✛

star fruit

The exotic star fruit lives up to its name thanks to its powerful antioxidant properties.

NUTRIENTS
Vitamin C, beta-carotene, folic acid; potassium

Also known as the star apple or carambola, the star fruit is completely edible: as well as the small soft seeds found inside, the external skin can be washed and eaten, too.

STAR FRUIT FACTS
*The star fruit originates from Sri Lanka.

*Harvested when green, the star fruit gradually turn a bright yellow, then a darker shade with brown tips when stored. This signals optimal ripeness, but doesn't impair texture or nutritional value.

*Anyone with kidney problems should avoid star fruit because of its oxalic acid content.

*In Chinese medicine, star fruit is known for its diuretic properties.

*In the Philippines, star fruit is eaten sprinkled with a little salt.

BOOSTS IMMUNITY
Nutritionally, the star fruit is a good source of disease-fighting beta-carotene. It is also packed with vitamin C, important for serious athletes because the body releases stress hormones into the bloodstream during heavy training, which can temporarily

---

SWEET AND SOUR NOODLES

300g/10½oz egg noodles
2 tbsp sesame oil
500g/1lb 2oz cooked prawns,
  shelled and deveined
4 small star fruit, sliced
  and tips removed
1 tbsp soy sauce
juice and zest of 1 lime
	Cook the noodles according to the packet instructions, then drain. Meanwhile, heat the oil in a pan until hot. Add the prawns, star fruit, and soy sauce and stir-fry 3 minutes. Toss with the noodles and lime juice and zest, and serve.

suppress the immune system. Eating vitamin-C-rich foods counteracts this by significantly raising antioxidant levels.

CORRECTS FLUID RETENTION
Star fruit also contains potassium, which has a mild diuretic effect, promoting the elimination of excess water.

Star fruit bruises easily and needs very careful handling.

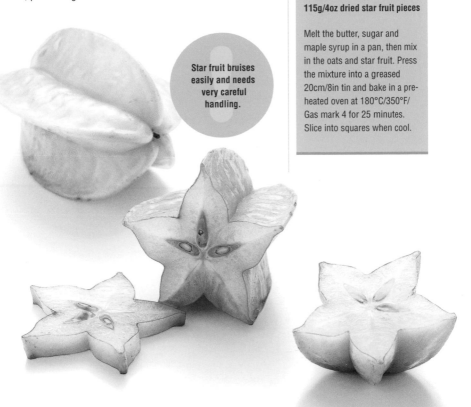

TROPICAL FLAPJACKS

175g/6oz butter
100g/3½oz/½ cup soft
   brown sugar
5 tbsp maple syrup
225g/8oz/2¼ cups rolled oats
115g/4oz dried star fruit pieces

Melt the butter, sugar and maple syrup in a pan, then mix in the oats and star fruit. Press the mixture into a greased 20cm/8in tin and bake in a pre-heated oven at 180°C/350°F/ Gas mark 4 for 25 minutes. Slice into squares when cool.

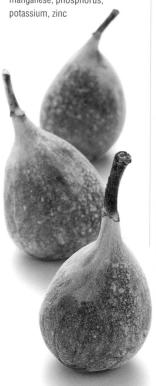

fig

Among the best plant sources of calcium, figs are known as the bone-friendly fruit.

NUTRIENTS
Vitamins B3, B5, B6, C, beta-carotene, folic acid; calcium, copper, iodine, iron, magnesium, manganese, phosphorus, potassium, zinc

Calcium is vital for strong bone density and particularly important for female athletes who train at high intensity. This is because they may experience low oestrogen levels and amenorrhoea, which can increase bone loss and the need for calcium. Dried figs offer a concentrated burst of simple carbohydrate for instant energy, while fresh figs provide a unique, sweet taste and crunchy texture, and a higher dose of the vital antioxidant vitamin C.

BAKED FIGS

12 figs, stems trimmed
6 tbsp maple syrup
100g/3½oz/½ cup
    walnut pieces
1 tsp ground cinnamon

Cut a cross in the top of each fig and squeeze the fruit open. Place them in a greased ovenproof dish and drizzle over the maple syrup. Sprinkle over the walnut pieces and cinnamon. Bake in a pre-heated oven at 180°C/350°F/Gas mark 4 for 15 minutes until soft. Serve immediately.

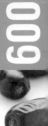

date

Chewy, dried dates make excellent "survival food" on long bike rides or when hiking.

NUTRIENTS
Vitamins B3, B5, B6, C, K, beta-carotene, folic acid; calcium, copper, iodine, iron, magnesium, manganese, phosphorus, potassium, selenium, zinc

The ideal preparation for exercise is to eat a light meal three hours before you begin, and then to top up with a snack just half an hour before. Dates are the perfect snack option – they're high in carbohydrates for energy and an excellent source of potassium, which is important for maintaining the fluid and electrolyte balances in the body.

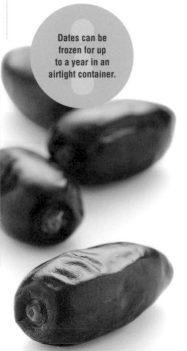

Dates can be frozen for up to a year in an airtight container.

FRUIT SQUARES

115g/4oz/⅔ cup dried dates
115g/4oz/⅔ cup dried apricots
125ml/4fl oz/½ cup lime juice
250g/9oz/2 cups self-raising flour
100g/3½oz/½ cup caster sugar
3 eggs, beaten

Blend the dates, apricots and lime juice in a food processor. Mix in the flour, sugar and eggs. Spoon the mixture into a greased 18cm/7in square cake tin. Bake in a pre-heated oven at 180°C/350°F/Gas mark 4 for 30–35 minutes. Allow to cool, then cut into squares.

mango

NUTRIENTS
Vitamins B3, C, E, beta-carotene; potassium

This sweet, juicy fruit provides an excellent vitamin boost and replaces essential minerals lost during a workout or match.

One serving (100g/3½oz) of mango provides 60 per cent of your daily vitamin-C needs, which helps the body to heal faster from the aches, pains, bumps and bruises that are often inevitable as a result of playing sport. Mango is a good source of potassium, which is important for maintaining normal blood pressure. It is also one of the few fruit sources of vitamin E, shown to help speed up post-exercise recovery rates.

TROPICAL FRUIT SLUSH
serves 2

**10 ice cubes
1 mango, peeled and
   roughly chopped
½ pineapple, peeled, cored
   and roughly chopped
10 strawberries, hulled
juice and zest of 1 lime**

Whizz the ice cubes in a blender until slushy. Add the mango, pineapple, strawberries, lime juice and zest and blend until smooth. Serve and drink immediately.

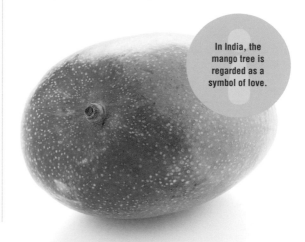

In India, the mango tree is regarded as a symbol of love.

papaya

A daily portion of tropical papaya can help to prevent "stitch", a sharp cramp in the side that can occur during exercise.

Also known as paw-paws, papayas are packed with anti-inflammatory vitamin C, which helps to soothe overworked body tissues. They are rich in potassium, which is important for good fluid balance, and muscle and nerve function. Papaya also contain papain, a potent enzyme that encourages the elimination of waste products and reduces the risk of exercise-related stomach cramps.

NUTRIENTS
Vitamins B3, B5, C, beta-carotene, folic acid; calcium, iodine, iron, magnesium, manganese, phosphorus, potassium, selenium, zinc

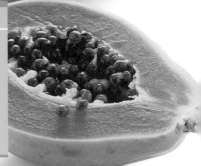

THAI-INSPIRED SALAD

2 papaya, peeled and
  deseeded
1 red pepper, deseeded
8 spring onions, chopped
100g/3½oz beansprouts
1 tbsp sugar
1 tbsp lime juice

1 tbsp fish sauce
a large handful mint, chopped

Dice the papaya and red pepper into 1cm/½in cubes. Toss all the ingredients in a large bowl, mixing well, and serve.

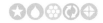

guava

NUTRIENTS
Vitamins B3, B5, B6, C, E,
beta-carotene, folic acid; calcium,
copper, iodine, iron, magnesium,
manganese, phosphorus,
potassium, selenium, zinc

The sweet-scented, creamy flesh of the exotic guava makes it an ideal addition to a pre- or post-exercise smoothie.

With four times the vitamin C and 70 times the fibre content of an orange, the guava is a nutritional powerhouse that can help to bolster the immune system. This is particularly important for regular exercisers, who use up their antioxidant reserves faster than non-exercisers. It is thought that the high fibre content of guavas lowers blood cholesterol by binding to it and eliminating it from the body.

GUAVA COULIS

12 guavas, cut in half
115g/4oz/½ cup icing sugar
125ml/4fl oz/½ cup lime juice
½ tsp vanilla extract

Simmer the guavas in 250ml/9fl oz/1 cup water for 8 minutes. Leave to cool, then push through a sieve into a bowl with the back of a spoon; discard the seeds. Place the pulp in a large pan, add the sugar, lime juice and vanilla extract. Bring to the boil, reduce the heat and simmer for 10 minutes until thickened.

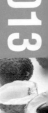

013

lychee

Light, rich in quick-energy carbohydrate and easily digestible, lychees make an exotic change from other fruit-bowl favourites.

NUTRIENTS
Vitamins B1, B2, C; copper, potassium

Deliciously refreshing lychees are the perfect nutritious snack to have before exercise or between training sessions. Available fresh, dried or tinned, nine lychees provide an adult's recommended daily intake of vitamin C and 15 per cent more polyphenols (which research shows help to keep the heart strong) than the equivalent number of grapes. To open a fresh lychee, score down one side with a sharp knife, peel off the crocodile-like skin and lift out the transparent, juicy flesh.

Lychees are native to China, the Philippines and India.

LYCHEE JELLY

8 lychees, peeled, pitted and halved
½ mango, peeled and cubed
55g/2oz/¼ cup caster sugar
2 x 11g/¼oz sachets powdered gelatine
500ml/17fl oz/2 cups apple juice

Place the lychees and mango in the bottom of 4 small jelly moulds or serving bowls. Heat the sugar in half the apple juice over a low heat until dissolved, then add the gelatine. Add the rest of the juice, pour over the fruit and refrigerate overnight. Tip out onto plates to serve.

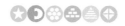

goji berry

Runners often nibble on dried goji berries to boost energy levels that may be diminishing.

Research shows that exercise increases the need for anti-oxidants, so goji berries are a great choice for athletes because they're rich in phytonutrients with significant antioxidant properties. Goji berries are also one of the few fruit sources of omega-3 and -6 essential fatty acids, good for keeping joints oiled. They are rich in amino acids to help to improve stamina, and betaine, a complex phytonutrient used by the liver to produce choline – a compound that promotes muscle growth.

SWEET POTATO AND GOJI BERRY FRITTERS

115g/4oz dried goji berries
2 sweet potatoes, peeled
1 apple, peeled and grated
115g/4oz/1 cup self-raising flour
2 eggs, separated
1 litre/35fl oz/4 cups sunflower oil, for frying

Soak the goji berries in water. Chop the potatoes into 2.5cm/1in cubes, boil for 10 minutes, drain and mash. Mix the mash, berries, apple, flour and egg yolks. Beat the egg whites until stiff and fold in. Deep-fry dollops in hot oil for 8–10 minutes. Drain and serve.

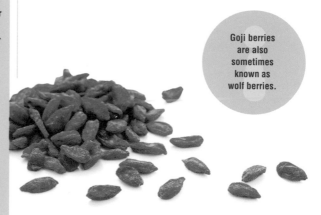

Goji berries are also sometimes known as wolf berries.

015

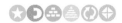

avocado

Add this nutrient-packed fruit to salads or spread on bread to help boost strength and endurance.

A good source of healthy monounsaturated fat and loaded with 20 vitamins, minerals and phytonutrients, avocados count among nature's true superfoods for anyone aiming to get fit. They contain more protein than any other fruit, making them great for strength and endurance. Just one avocado provides half the recommended daily intake of vitamin B6 – essential for helping the body to release energy from food.

NUTRIENTS
Vitamins B1, B2, B5, B6, C, E, K, folic acid; copper, iron, phosphorus, potassium, zinc; carotenoids; monounsaturated fats

TANGY SUMMER SALAD

3 tbsp olive oil
1 tsp clear honey
1 red onion, grated
1 tsp Dijon mustard
4 ripe avocados, peeled, pitted and sliced
1 pink grapefruit, peeled and segmented
a large handful rocket leaves

Whisk the oil, honey, onion and mustard together in a bowl. Add the avocados, grapefruit and rocket, toss well in the dressing and serve.

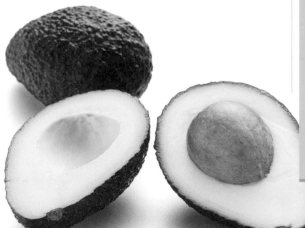

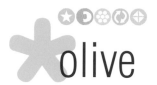

olive

NUTRIENTS

Vitamins E, K, beta-carotene; calcium, copper, iodine, iron, magnesium, manganese, phosphorus, potassium, selenium, zinc; omega-9 essential fatty acids

OLIVE FACTS

*The oil made from olives is one of the healthiest culinary oils as it contains lots of monounsaturates, which are good for the heart.

*Olive oil is available in a variety of grades, which reflect the degree to which it has been processed. "Extra virgin" is the best choice, as it retains the most antioxidants.

*Store olives and olive oils in opaque tubs and dark, tinted bottles, as these will help to prevent the harmful oxidation caused by exposure to light.

Staples of Mediterranean cuisine, olives are bursting with health benefits for fitness fanatics.

There are hundreds of olive varieties. In general, black varieties are moist and full flavoured, while green have a milder taste.

BEST FOR THE HEART

Olives are thought to keep the heart healthy because they're among the best sources of monounsaturated fats, which help to lower harmfully high cholesterol levels.

PROTECTS JOINTS

Super-rich in vitamin E and omega-9 fatty acids, which have anti-inflammatory properties, olives also help to protect the

OLIVE AND NUT DIP

225g/8oz pitted green olives	Whizz the olives, walnuts
100g/3½oz shelled walnuts	and pine nuts in a blender
55g/2oz pine nuts	until smooth. Mix in
2 tbsp grated Romano cheese	the grated cheese and
1 tbsp olive oil	olive oil. Serve with
breadsticks, to serve	breadsticks.

joints from workout wear and tear. In addition, the essential fatty acids in olives have been shown to boost the body's ability to remove unwanted stored fat in the cells.

STRENGTHENS BONES

One recent scientific study suggests that eating olives on a regular basis also plays an important role in protecting bones against osteoporosis.

MINI KEBABS
Makes 24

24 black olives, pitted
and halved
24 cherry tomatoes, halved
24 cubes feta cheese
48 basil leaves
black pepper

Spear 2 olive halves, 2 tomato halves, 2 basil leaves and a cube of cheese onto each of 24 cocktail sticks, alternating ingredients. Season, arrange on a serving dish and serve.

In the wild, olive trees bear fruit only every other year.

lettuce

NUTRIENTS

Vitamins B1, B3, B5, C, E, K, beta-carotene, folic acid; calcium, iodine, iron, magnesium, manganese, phosphorus, potassium, selenium, silica, zinc

A salad and sandwich staple, lettuce provides vital nutrients for helping the body to make energy.

Lettuce contains many minerals, including iron, calcium, magnesium and zinc, all of which help to generate energy. Equally important for an athlete's health is the folic acid content – this B-vitamin protects the heart by converting a damaging chemical called homocysteine into benign substances. If not converted, homocysteine can directly damage blood vessels, greatly increasing the risk of heart attack and stroke.

CHEESY GRILLED LETTUCE

1 Romaine lettuce
1 tbsp olive oil
200g/7oz Camembert
2 tsp balsamic vinegar

Cut the lettuce lengthways into quarters, brush with the oil and grill for 2 minutes on each side. Arrange in a shallow ovenproof dish, top with thin slices of cheese and drizzle over the vinegar. Bake in a pre-heated oven at 220°C/425°F/Gas mark 7 for 5 minutes until the cheese is bubbling, then serve.

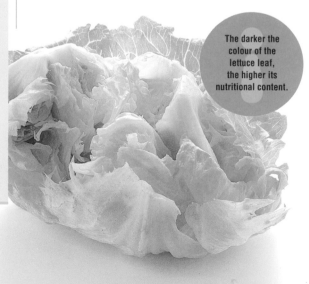

The darker the colour of the lettuce leaf, the higher its nutritional content.

pepper

Whether eaten raw as a crunchy crudité or softened in a stir-fry or roasting dish, sweet peppers pack a powerful nutritional punch.

After exercise, the body continues to burn fat. Peppers mirror this process because they contain substances that significantly increase heat production in the body for more than 20 minutes after they are eaten, helping to burn calories quicker. One 150g/5½oz serving of pepper provides the daily recommended intake of vitamin C and beta-carotene, which both have potent immunity-boosting antioxidant properties.

NUTRIENTS
Vitamins B3, B6, C, E, K, beta-carotene, biotin, folic acid; calcium, iodine, iron, magnesium, manganese, phosphorus, potassium, zinc

RED PEPPER SALSA

1 red pepper, deseeded
  and finely diced
2 beef tomatoes, finely diced
½ small red pepper, deseeded
  and finely chopped
1 small cucumber, finely diced
4 tbsp chopped coriander
juice and zest of ½ lime

Mix the ingredients together in a bowl. Serve as a dip or a sauce.

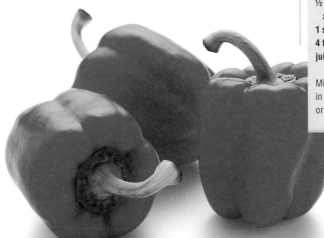

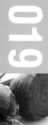

beetroot

NUTRIENTS
Vitamins B3, B5, C, folic acid,
beta-carotene; calcium, iodine,
iron, magnesium, manganese,
phosphorus, potassium, zinc

A high natural sugar content helps beetroot to revive flagging energy levels on the playing field.

Not only does beetroot provide easily digestible sugars, but its dietary fibre also slows down the absorption of these carbohydrates into the blood, which means the body is supplied with a steady stream of energy. Beetroot juice is a concentrated source of the antioxidant betacyanin and, if drunk on an empty stomach, is an effective internal cleanser. Other great ways to introduce this vegetable into the diet include grating it raw into salads or adding chunks to slow-cooking soups and stews.

RAINBOW ROOT SALAD

2 large beetroot,
  peeled and grated
3 carrots, peeled
  and grated
1 parsnip, peeled and grated
1 red onion, grated
juice of 1 lemon
1 tbsp olive oil

Mix the grated vegetables well in a large bowl. Drizzle over the lemon juice and oil, then serve.

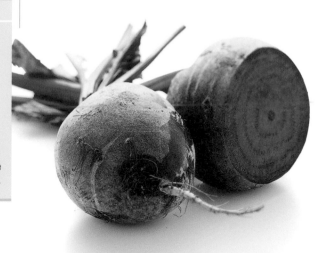

020

onion

Famed for adding flavour to savoury recipes, onions boast incredible fitness benefits, too.

For anyone aiming to reach peak physical fitness, onions can offer several minerals, including chromium, manganese and potassium, which help to break down fat deposits and speed up metabolism. They are also full of quercetin (a flavonoid that is not destroyed during the cooking process), which has been shown to reduce fatigue. Studies suggest that onions can help to maintain healthy bones by inhibiting the activity of osteoclasts – the cells that break down bone.

NUTRIENTS
Vitamins B6, C, folic acid; chromium, copper, manganese, phosphorus, potassium

Onions contain sulphurous amino acids that boost the body's ability to detoxify.

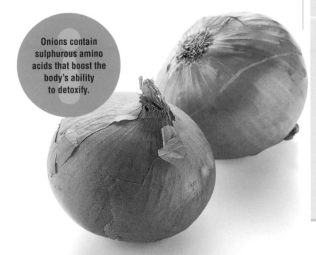

CARAMELIZED ONION SAUCE

4 large onions, chopped
1 garlic clove, crushed
2 tbsp olive oil
1 tsp Dijon mustard
250ml/9fl oz/1 cup
    single cream

Cook the onions and garlic in the oil in a pan for 45 minutes on a very low heat. Stir in the mustard and cook for a further 10 minutes. Then, stir in the cream and serve.

pea

NUTRIENTS
Vitamins B-complex, C, K, beta-carotene, folic acid; copper, iron, magnesium, manganese, phosphorus, potassium, zinc

For weight-conscious sports players, peas are an excellent, quick-to-cook side dish.

Exceptionally rich in both soluble and insoluble fibre, peas are one of nature's best aids to weight control. Studies demonstrate that the more fibre we consume, the less likely we are to gain weight and the more readily we shed excess fat. Fibre has also been shown to have a positive effect on the hormones in the intestines that control appetite. In addition, the vitamin C and iron in peas help to keep energy levels topped up.

PEA RISOTTO

1 onion, finely chopped
1 tbsp olive oil
300g/10½oz/2 cups peas
175g/6oz/¾ cup Arborio rice
250ml/9fl oz/1 cup milk
750ml/26fl oz/3 cups hot
   vegetable stock
a handful mint, chopped
55g/2oz Parmesan, grated

In a heavy-bottomed pan, fry the onion in the oil until soft. Add the peas and cook for 2 minutes. Stir in the rice and milk. Gradually add the stock one ladle at a time, stirring until absorbed. Cook for 20 minutes. Then, gently stir in the mint, sprinkle the cheese over the top and serve.

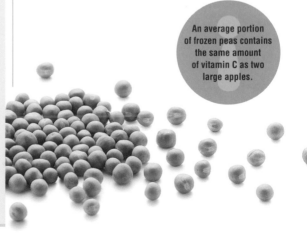

An average portion of frozen peas contains the same amount of vitamin C as two large apples.

carrot

This versatile vegetable provides instant energy, fibre and a long list of health-boosting nutrients.

The highly concentrated sugars in carrots are easily absorbed for on-the-spot energy. Carrots are among the richest sources of beta-carotene, which is converted by the body into the antioxidant vitamin A to help to prevent heart disease and speed up post-exercise recovery time. Eating two carrots a day can help to reduce high cholesterol levels. Nibble on raw sticks, drink the juice, chop into stews and soups or grate into cakes.

NUTRIENTS
Vitamin C, beta-carotene, biotin, folic acid; calcium, iron, magnesium, manganese, phosphorus, potassium; bioflavonoids; limonin; lycopene

CARROT CAKE

115g/4oz butter
115g/4oz/½ cup clear honey
115g/4oz/½ cup brown sugar
225g/8oz/1⅔ cups wholemeal flour
1 tsp baking powder
225g/8oz carrots, peeled and grated
1 tsp ground cinnamon

Grease a 20-cm/8-in round cake tin. In a bowl, beat the butter, honey and sugar. Fold in the remaining ingredients and spoon into the tin. Bake in a pre-heated oven at 180°C/350°F/Gas mark 4 for 1 hour.

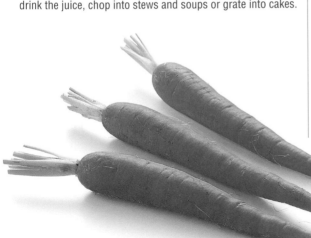

butternut squash

NUTRIENTS
Vitamins B1, B3, B5, B6, C,
E, K, beta-carotene, folic acid;
calcium, copper, iron, magnesium,
phosphorus, potassium,
selenium, zinc

Squash is a nutritional winner and is delicious in soups and stews and with other roasted vegetables.

BOOSTS IMMUNITY

Like all orange fruit and vegetables, the butternut squash is a great source of beta-carotene, which the body converts to vitamin A, needed for a healthy immune system and good digestive and respiratory-tract function.

You can tell if a squash is ripe by tapping it – if ripe, it will sound hollow.

SPICY ROASTED VEGETABLES

3 tbsp sunflower seeds
1 tsp chilli powder
1 tsp cumin seeds
1 tsp ground coriander
1 tsp ground ginger
1 butternut squash, peeled
  and deseeded
2 courgettes, chopped
1 red pepper, deseeded
  and sliced
200g/7oz button mushrooms
3 tbsp olive oil
1 tbsp balsamic vinegar

Toast the sunflower seeds and spices in a frying pan over a low heat for 3 minutes. Chop the squash into 5cm/2in chunks. Place the squash and the other vegetables in an ovenproof dish. Add the oil, balsamic vinegar, seeds and spices, and mix well together. Bake in a pre-heated oven at 190°C/ 375°F/Gas mark 5 for 1 hour, stirring occasionally, then serve.

SUSTAINS ENERGY

A great provider of energy-sustaining carbohydrates, squash contains high levels of the minerals potassium and magnesium, which help to maintain efficient energy production. A lack of these minerals can lead to fatigue, muscle cramps and an increased risk of high cholesterol, high blood pressure and heart problems. Squashes are also thought to reduce the symptoms of prostatic hyperplasia, a benign prostate condition.

BUTTERNUT SQUASH FACTS

*Archaeologists have found evidence in Mexican caves to suggest that humankind has been eating squash for at least 7,000 years.

*Butternut squash is a variety of winter squash. Other varieties include acorn, spaghetti and sweet squash.

*Winter squash develops more beta-carotene after being stored than it contains immediately after picking.

*The smallest butternut squashes are usually the tastiest.

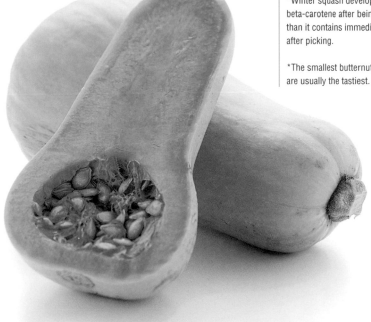

cauliflower

NUTRIENTS
Vitamins B3, B5, B6, C, folic acid; calcium, manganese, potassium, zinc

Prevent a sluggish system slowing you down with this excellent internal cleanser.

A member of the nutritionally powerful cruciferous family of vegetables, cauliflower contains a compound called glucosinolate, which fuels and strengthens the liver in its job as a detoxifier, cleansing the body for peak performance. Cauliflower is also a good source of the B-vitamins, the most important nutrients needed for energy production and to support the adrenal glands.

CURRIED CAULIFLOWER AND LENTILS

1 tbsp olive oil
1 garlic clove, crushed
1 onion, finely chopped
1 tbsp curry powder
250ml/9fl oz/1 cup hot vegetable stock
1 cauliflower, broken into florets
115g/4oz/½ cup red lentils
brown rice, to serve

Gently heat the oil in a large pan. Add the garlic, onion and curry powder and fry until soft. Stir in the stock, cauliflower and lentils, cover and simmer for about 20 minutes. Serve with brown rice.

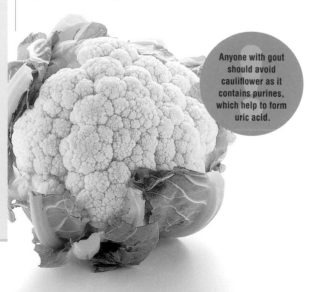

Anyone with gout should avoid cauliflower as it contains purines, which help to form uric acid.

025

broccoli

Celebrated as a superfood, broccoli contains compounds that can boost motivation, helping to lift a fatigue-related mood dip.

The long list of nutrients in broccoli means that it is a brilliant energy-reviver. The zinc enhances mental alertness, vitamin B5 helps the body to metabolize fats into energy and the folic acid encourages the production of serotonin, a mood-lifting chemical in the brain. A good plant source of calcium, broccoli also promotes post-workout muscle relaxation and has bone-building properties.

NUTRIENTS
Vitamins B1, B3, B5, B6, C, E, K, beta-carotene, folic acid; calcium, iodine, iron, magnesium, manganese, phosphorus, potassium, zinc

SPICY BROCCOLI

2 heads of broccoli, broken into florets
1 onion, finely chopped
2 tbsp sunflower oil
1 tbsp curry powder
½ tsp chilli powder
250ml/9fl oz/1 cup single cream
55g/2oz flaked almonds

Steam the broccoli for 6–8 minutes until tender. In another pan, fry the onion in the oil until soft. Add the broccoli, spices and cream, and simmer for 5 minutes. Scatter over the almonds. Serve as a side dish.

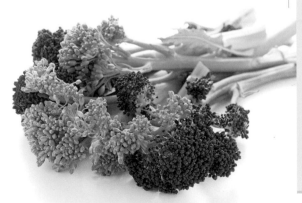

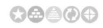

sweetcorn

Barbecued or boiled, sweetcorn is a crunchy and deliciously sweet accompaniment to meat.

Sweetcorn, made up of the yellow or white kernels that grow on the cob, is the most nutritious way to eat corn, as it provides starchy carbohydrates and a vegetable source of protein for a steady stream of energy during exercise. Yellow sweetcorn is a good source of the potent antioxidant lutein, which promotes healthy vision and a strong cardiovascular system. When tinned or frozen, sweetcorn retains most of its goodness.

SWEETCORN RELISH

2 corn on the cob
55g/2oz butter
1 red pepper, deseeded
and finely diced
1 red onion, finely diced
2 celery stalks, finely diced
½ cucumber, finely diced

Boil the corn in a large pan of salted water for 7–8 minutes until tender. Drain, slice off the kernels and mix with the butter. Mix well with the remaining ingredients.

To stop corn burning on a barbecue, soak it in water for 10 minutes and wrap in foil before cooking.

chard

Eaten raw or cooked like spinach, chard is a valuable source of iron for non-meat-eating athletes.

A member of the beet family, chard has crunchy stalks and spinach-like leaves with a slightly bitter, earthy flavour. Chard is an excellent bone-builder thanks to its calcium, magnesium and vitamin-K content, which are all thought to aid bone mineralization. Many of the nutrients in chard keep blood vessels strong, allowing blood to move oxygen around the body easily to boost strength and energy levels.

NUTRIENTS
Vitamins C, K, beta-carotene, folic acid; calcium, iron, magnesium, zinc

CHARD WITH SESAME SEEDS

1 onion, finely chopped
1 tbsp olive oil
1 tbsp tamari sauce
55g/2oz/⅓ cup sesame seeds
300g/10½oz chard leaves

In a pan, fry the onion in the oil until soft. Stir in the tamari sauce and sesame seeds. Chop the chard leaves into slices, add to the pan and stir until wilted. Serve immediately.

pak choi

Crank up the nutritional content of stir-fries and spring rolls with this potent Chinese vegetable.

NUTRIENTS
Vitamins B2, B6, C, beta-carotene, folic acid; calcium, iron, magnesium, manganese, phosphorus, potassium, selenium, zinc

Pak choi belongs to the cabbage family and has a mild, mustardy taste. Both the leaves and stalks are edible and packed with nutrients. Baby leaves with very fine stalks work brilliantly in salads. One average portion of cooked pak choi contains the same amount of calcium as 125ml/4fl oz/½ cup of full-fat milk. Pak choi also has an abundance of vitamin C, which aids recovery from sports injuries by strengthening cell walls.

CRUNCHY VEGETABLE STIR-FRY

1 tbsp sesame oil
1 onion, finely chopped
1 garlic clove, crushed
½ cabbage, shredded
150g/5½ oz mushrooms, sliced
4 pak choi stalks, shredded

Heat the oil in a wok over a high heat. Add the onion and garlic and stir-fry for 2 minutes. Add the cabbage, mushrooms and pak choi and stir-fry for a further 4 minutes. Serve immediately.

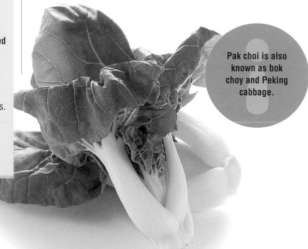

Pak choi is also known as bok choy and Peking cabbage.

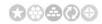

mushroom

Sugar cravings, whether they occur before, during or after exercise, can be tamed by including mushrooms regularly on the menu.

Mushrooms are a slow-release energy food, thanks to their high content of vegetable protein. They're also especially rich in chromium, which helps to stabilize blood-sugar levels and, in turn, helps to control sugar cravings. The older you are, the less likely you are to be taking in enough chromium. Mushrooms are also an important source of vitamin B12 for vegetarians, which is vital for maintaining healthy energy levels.

NUTRIENTS
Vitamins B1, B2, B3, B5, B6, B12, E, folic acid; calcium, chromium, copper, iron, manganese, phosphorus, potassium, selenium, zinc

MUSHROOM PÂTÉ

375g/13oz chestnut mushrooms, chopped
2 tbsp olive oil
1 tbsp soy sauce
200g/7oz mascapone
2 tbsp chopped tarragon

In a pan, fry the mushrooms in the oil for 2 minutes. Add 4 tablespoons of water and simmer for 10 minutes. Allow to cool, then drain and purée in a blender. Stir in the remaining ingredients. Refrigerate for at least 1 hour, then serve.

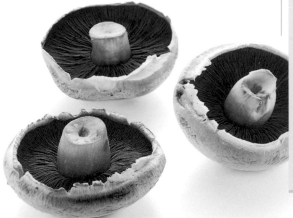

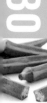

okra

NUTRIENTS
Vitamins B1, B3, B5, B6, C, K, beta-carotene, folic acid; calcium, iodine, iron, magnesium, manganese, phosphorus, potassium, selenium, zinc

If training is disrupted due to an upset stomach, okra can help the digestive system to recover.

This vegetable, which looks like a mini green banana, is a staple in Middle Eastern cooking and regularly features in Indian, North African and Caribbean cuisine. Okra is a good source of soluble fibre, which helps to reduce cholesterol and stabilize blood sugar levels. It also contains psyllium, which acts as a probiotic in the gut, encouraging the growth of friendly bacteria and helping to soothe stomach upsets.

VEGETABLE GUMBO

400g/14oz okra, stems removed
2 courgettes, ends trimmed
2 yellow peppers, deseeded
3 beef tomatoes
1 onion, finely chopped
1 tbsp sunflower oil
1 tbsp tomato purée
brown rice, to serve

Chop the vegetables into 2.5cm/1in cubes. In an oven-proof dish, fry the onion, then the vegetables, in the oil until soft. Mix in the purée, cover and bake in a pre-heated oven at 190°C/375°F/Gas mark 5 for 1 hour. Serve with brown rice.

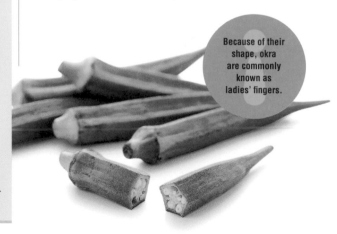

Because of their shape, okra are commonly known as ladies' fingers.

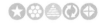

sweet potato

An oven-baked sweet potato is the perfect light meal for anyone who prefers the gym to the kitchen.

Despite its sweet taste, this root vegetable provides healthy complex carbohydrate, releasing a steady stream of energy into the bloodstream and helping to regulate blood-sugar levels. An antioxidant powerhouse, sweet potato is an excellent source of vitamins C, E and beta-carotene, which work synergistically with one another to ward off post-workout fatigue. It also contains vitamin B6 to help to protect the heart.

NUTRIENTS
Vitamins B1, B3, B5, B6, C, E, beta-carotene, folic acid; calcium, iodine, iron, magnesium, manganese, phosphorus, potassium, selenium, zinc

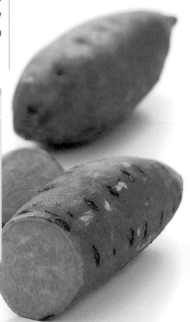

STEAMED SWEET POTATOES AND MANGETOUTS

3 sweet potatoes, peeled and cubed
100g/3½oz mangetout
3 tbsp soy sauce
1 tbsp sunflower seeds

Chop the sweet potatoes into 2.5cm/1in slices and place them in a large casserole dish.

Add 2 tablespoons of water, cover and steam for 8 minutes until tender. Stir in the mangetout and cook for a further 2 minutes. Transfer the vegetables to a bowl, and sprinkle over the soy sauce and the sunflower seeds. Serve as a side dish or a snack.

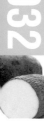

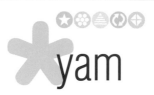

yam

NUTRIENTS
Vitamins B1, B3, B5, B6, C,
E, folic acid; calcium, iodine,
iron, magnesium, manganese,
phosphorus, potassium,
selenium, zinc

YAM FACTS
*One of the most widely consumed
foods in the world, yams have been
cultivated since 8,000BCE in Africa
and Asia.

*Yams come in yellow, white,
ivory and purple varieties.

*There are more than 200
species of yam.

*Yams sometimes have offshoots,
known as "toes".

*Unlike sweet potatoes, yams are
toxic if eaten raw, although both are
perfectly safe to eat when cooked.

A fabulous form of slow-releasing energy, this
starchy root vegetable is a more fitness-friendly
alternative to the potato.

Thanks to their rich fibre content, yams rank lower on the
glycaemic index and provide a more sustained form of
carbohydrate energy than the more popular potatoes.

BOOSTS ENERGY
High in potassium and low in sodium, yams help to regulate
the fluid balance that exercise can so easily deplete through
perspiration. Yam contains several of the B-vitamins and is

CITRUS YAMS	
2 yams, peeled and chopped into 2.5cm/1in chunks 4 tbsp olive oil 1 tbsp chopped parsley 1 tbsp chopped coriander juice and grated zest of 1 orange juice and zest of 1 lime	Steam the yam for 20 minutes until tender. In a bowl, whisk together the oil, parsley, coriander, juice and zest of the orange and lime. Fold the cooked yam into the dressing. Serve as a starter, a side-dish or a snack.

particularly rich in vitamin B1, useful for boosting energy levels, and manganese, a trace mineral that helps the body with the metabolism of carbohydrates.

BALANCES BLOOD SUGAR AND SALT

Discoretine, another chemical found in yam, is particularly useful for athletes, as it reduces blood sugar and increases blood flow through the kidneys. This promotes the excretion of excess salt, which in turn helps to reduce high blood pressure.

Never try to eat the skin of a yam, as it is woody and inedible.

YAM DUMPLINGS ROLLED IN POPPY SEEDS

1 yam, peeled and chopped
3 egg yolks
½ tsp chilli powder
1 tsp cornflour
3 tbsp self-raising flour
4 tbsp poppy seeds

Boil the yam for 20 minutes until tender. Drain, allow to cool, then purée in a food processor. Transfer to a bowl and mix in the egg yolks, chilli and flours. Form into balls and roll in the poppy seeds. Line a steamer with foil, place over a pan of simmering water. Steam for 10 minutes and serve.

033

aubergine

NUTRIENTS
Vitamins B1, B3, B6, C, K, beta-carotene, folic acid; calcium, copper, iodine, iron, magnesium, manganese, phosphorus, potassium, selenium, zinc

Thanks to its high number of healing compounds, aubergine helps to ward off many performance-impairing illnesses.

Aubergines are loaded with antioxidants, including chlorogenic acid, which is anti-viral, anti-bacterial and anti-fungal, and nasunin, a flavonoid found to mop up free radicals, protecting the body against diseases. A member of the nightshade family, aubergines should be avoided by sufferers of osteoarthritis as they may increase inflammation in the joints.

AUBERGINE AND RICOTTA ROLLS

1 large aubergine,
  ends trimmed
3 tbsp olive oil
juice and zest of 1 lemon
200g/7oz ricotta cheese
4 sun-dried tomatoes,
  chopped
black pepper

Cut the aubergine lengthways into 5mm/¼in thick slices. Cover with the oil and lemon juice and zest. Place on a baking tray and grill for 3 minutes on each side. Put some cheese, tomato and black pepper on each slice. Fold and secure with a cocktail stick. Grill for 2 minutes, then serve.

vine leaves

Commonly used in Greek cuisine, vine leaves contain flavonoid antioxidants to help to prevent post-exercise muscle soreness.

Tender, dark green vine leaves, with a subtle flavour and texture similar to spinach, are available fresh and ready-to-use in salt-water pouches. Like all leafy green vegetables, they contain flavonoids and vitamin C, useful for anyone working out regularly because a diet rich in antioxidants has been shown to promote faster recovery after exercise and to help the body stay in peak condition.

NUTRIENTS
Vitamin C, E, K; calcium, iron, magnesium, manganese, phosphorus, potassium, selenium, sodium, zinc

STUFFED VINE LEAVES

400g/14oz minced lamb
200g/7oz/1 cup long-grain rice
a handful mint, chopped
1 tbsp olive oil
3 spring onions, finely chopped
salt and black pepper
16 vine leaves

Mix the lamb, rice, mint, oil and spring onions in a bowl, and season. Place 2 vine leaves on top of each other, add a dollop of the mixture and roll up to form a parcel. Repeat to make 8 parcels. Place in a steamer over a pan of simmering water. Steam the parcels for 1 hour or until the leaves are tender, and the meat and rice are cooked. Serve 2 parcels each as a starter.

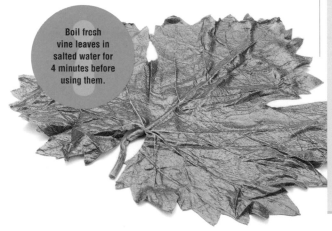

Boil fresh vine leaves in salted water for 4 minutes before using them.

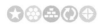

crayfish

Freshwater crustaceans, crayfish are loaded with immunity-boosting minerals.

Crayfish look like miniature versions of lobsters, to which they are closely related. They are an excellent source of selenium, an antioxidant mineral that research shows is one of the best natural cell-protectors around, as it mops up the free radicals produced by the body during exercise. A selenium deficiency is associated with anxiety, depression and fatigue. Crayfish is also a valuable source of zinc, which helps to ward off disease.

CRAYFISH TAGLIATELLE

300g/10½oz fresh tagliatelle
500g/1lb 2oz cherry tomatoes,
  halved
1 tbsp olive oil
juice and zest of 1 lemon
400g/14oz cooked crayfish tails
a handful basil leaves

Cook the tagliatelle in a large pan of salted, boiling water for 6–8 minutes or as instructed on the package, then drain. In another pan, sauté the tomatoes in the oil for 3 minutes. Add the lemon juice and zest, crayfish, basil and tagliatelle, and serve.

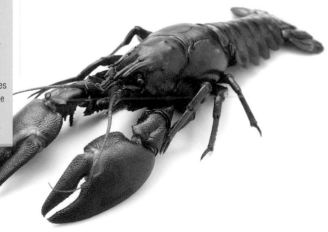

036

trout

With a third of the fat of salmon, trout is an excellent alternative for the calorie-conscious.

Trout is a good source of essential fatty acids, which have been found to help increase an athlete's speed, because they improve the delivery of oxygen to the body's cells, boosting energy levels and building stamina. Omega-3 fats have also been found to stimulate production of a hormone called leptin, which helps to control appetite. In addition, trout is packed with protein to encourage muscle growth and repair.

NUTRIENTS
Vitamins A, B1, B2, B6, B12; calcium, iron, selenium; omega-3 essential fatty acids

TROUT STUFFED WITH SAGE AND ROSEMARY

4 fresh whole trout,
   gutted and cleaned
a handful sage
a handful rosemary
juice of 2 lemons
55g/2oz butter
steamed greens, to serve

Place the trout in an ovenproof dish. Stuff some herbs into each fish and drizzle with lemon juice. Melt the butter and pour over the fish. Bake in a pre-heated oven at 180°C/350°F/ Gas mark 4 for 35 minutes. Serve with steamed greens.

One 100g/3½oz portion of trout contains just 135 calories.

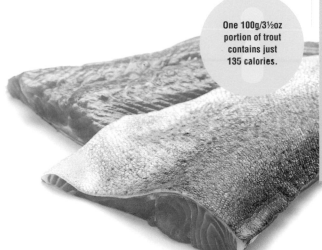

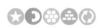

salmon

NUTRIENTS
Vitamins A, B3, B6, B12, D, E, folic acid; calcium, magnesium, phosphorus, selenium; omega-3 essential fatty acids

One of the healthiest forms of protein, bone-friendly salmon is a superb choice for athletes.

If regular exercisers are not getting enough protein in their diet, they take longer both to recover after training and to build up their muscles and stamina. Salmon provides plenty of protein, as well as one of the highest levels among all foods of omega-3 essential fatty acids and DHA (docosahexaenoic acid), both of which are renowned for helping to reduce post-exercise joint stiffness. DHA is especially important for helping blood to flow smoothly through the arteries.

SALMON PATTIES

85g/3oz/scant ½ cup
   long-grain rice
1 egg
1 garlic clove
1 onion, halved
2 tsp sunflower oil, plus
   extra for frying
500g/1lb 2oz salmon fillets,
   boned, skinned and chopped
1 tbsp chopped parsley

In a pan, bring 125ml/4½fl oz/ ½ cup water to the boil. Add the rice, reduce the heat and simmer for 10 minutes. Allow to cool. In a food processor, purée the egg, garlic, onion and oil. Mix well with the rice, salmon and parsley, and form into 8 patties. Fry in batches in the oil for 4–5 minutes on each side.

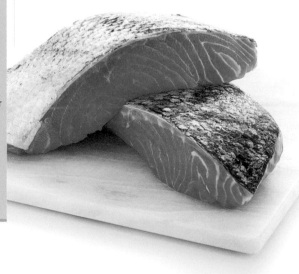

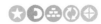

tuna

Tuna provides a low-fat, protein-packed nutritional hit that's quick to prepare.

Lean sources of protein are key for anyone who's physically active, as they prevent slumps in energy without sending calorie intake soaring. Like other oily fish, fresh tuna is exceptionally rich in omega-3 fatty acids, which play an important role in energy production and helping to burn excess fat. Flash-cook thin slices of tuna on a pre-heated ridged grill or, for an even speedier option, use tinned varieties.

NUTRIENTS
Vitamins B1, B3, B6, B12, D, E; iodine, magnesium, phosphorus, potassium, selenium, sodium; omega-3 essential fatty acids

Look out for albacore, skipjack and yellowfin tuna, which are the most nutritious kinds.

TUNA AND GREEN BEAN SALAD

115g/4oz steamed
  green beans, sliced
115g/4oz cherry tomatoes
2 tbsp olive oil
400g/14oz fresh tuna steaks

In a bowl, toss the beans with the tomatoes and oil. Grill the tuna for 3 minutes on each side. Slice, arrange over the salad and serve.

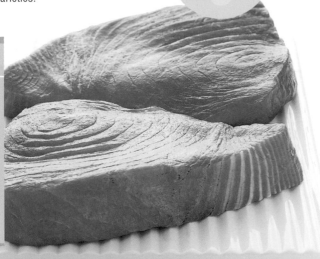

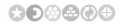

sardine

NUTRIENTS
Vitamins B3, B6, D, E; calcium, iodine, iron, potassium, selenium; omega-3 essential fatty acids

Being one of the few non-dairy sources of easily absorbable calcium makes sardines a first-rate food for athletes.

Including plenty of calcium in the diet is essential for strong bones and, according to research, can also help the body to burn body fat more efficiently. Sardines are packed with protein, iron, zinc, essential fatty acids and vitamin D, and are exceptionally rich in calcium. Ask the fishmonger to remove the heads and backbones, but leave the other bones – once cooked they're very soft and you can just mash them with a fork.

JAPANESE SARDINES

450g/1lb sardines,
 washed and dried
125ml/4fl oz/½ cup soy sauce
4 tbsp white wine vinegar
juice and zest of 1 lime
1 lemon grass stem,
 chopped
2.5cm/1in piece root ginger,
 peeled and chopped
2 garlic cloves, crushed
1 tsp chilli powder

Arrange the sardines in a shallow dish. Mix together the remaining ingredients in a bowl and pour over the sardines. Cover and refrigerate for 3 hours. Discard the marinade and grill the sardines for 3–5 minutes, turning once, until the flesh flakes.

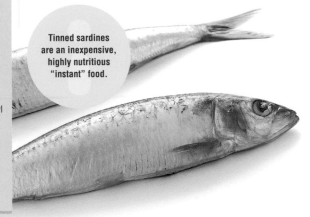

Tinned sardines are an inexpensive, highly nutritious "instant" food.

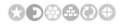

mackerel

Put fresh, smoked or tinned mackerel on the menu to guarantee a host of health and fitness benefits.

Mackerel fillets are simple to cook and easy to digest. They're loaded with omega-3 essential fatty acids, which help to prevent heart disease and keep joints healthy, while their vitamin-E content helps to protect the nerves and heart from the wear and tear of sport. Mackerel is also one of the few food sources of vitamin D (usually manufactured in the body from sunlight), which, along with the calcium, is crucial for good bone health.

NUTRIENTS
Vitamins B3, B6, B12, D, E, calcium, iodine, potassium, selenium; omega-3 essential fatty acids

MACKEREL MASH

4 potatoes, peeled
   and diced
25g/1oz butter
1 tbsp milk
1 tbsp chopped parsley
2 shallots, finely chopped
400g/14oz cooked mackerel,
   skinned and flaked
black pepper

Cook the potatoes in a large pan of boiling, salted water until soft. Mash with the butter and milk. Stir in the parsley, shallots and mackerel, and season with pepper.

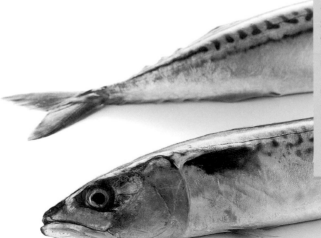

041

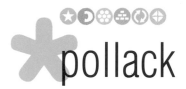

pollack

NUTRIENTS
Vitamins B3, B12; calcium, iodine, magnesium, potassium, selenium; omega-3 essential fatty acids

Pollack's firm, white, flaky flesh makes it a delicious, nutrient-packed substitute for cod.

As global stocks of cod become seriously depleted, pollack is rapidly becoming an increasingly popular alternative.

INCREASES ENERGY

One average portion of pollack provides more than 20 per cent of the recommended daily intake of energy-boosting selenium

Pollack is a prime low-fat source of protein, containing less than 5 per cent of fat in its flesh.

POLLACK CHOWDER

1 tbsp olive oil
1 onion, chopped
3 carrots, peeled
  and diced
2 large potatoes,
  peeled and diced
115g/4oz/½ cup brown rice
500ml/17fl oz/2 cups
  vegetable stock
500g/1lb 2oz pollack, boned,
  skinned and cut into chunks
4 tbsp milk

Heat the oil in a pan, add the onion and fry lightly. Add the carrots, potatoes, rice and stock. Bring to the boil, reduce the heat and simmer for 15 minutes. Add the fish chunks and milk, and simmer for a further 8 minutes. Serve immediately.

and vitamins B3 and B12, as well as more than 10 per cent of the recommended daily intake of magnesium and potassium, which balance the level of fluid in the body. Pollack is also rich in iodine, a mineral needed to regulate the metabolism and the activity of the thyroid gland.

REBUILDS MUSCLE

A fantastic source of lean protein, pollack helps the body to feel full for longer, especially when eaten with carbohydrate, such as brown rice. This combination also aids the repair of muscle because the carbohydrate triggers the release of the hormone insulin, which acts like a key, opening the cells to allow them to absorb the amino acids contained in the protein.

POLLACK FACTS

*When fresh, pollack never smells fishy, the eyes appear bright and clear, and the flesh "gives" slightly when pressed and then springs back into shape.

*To store pollack, remove the packaging, rinse under cold water, and pat dry with paper towels. Place on a cake rack in a shallow pan filled with crushed ice. Cover with cling film and set in the coldest part of the fridge.

*If it's well wrapped, pollack can be frozen for 3–4 months.

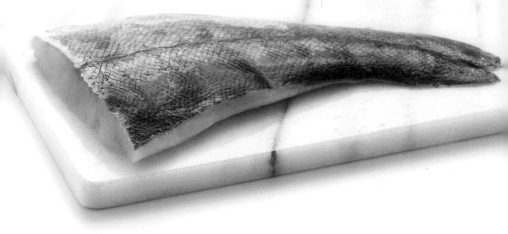

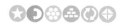

prawn

NUTRIENTS
Vitamins B3, B12; calcium,
iodine, magnesium, phosphorus,
potassium, selenium, sodium, zinc

The world's most popular and versatile crustaceans, prawns work well in sandwiches, salads, stir-fries and seafood stews.

Prawns are packed full of goodness, such as B-vitamins and many vital minerals, including potassium, magnesium and sodium, which all help to restore an athlete's electrolyte balance after a heavy training session. As prawns are higher in sodium than most foods (although not in harmful levels), they can also help to prevent the mineral imbalance that can result from drinking too much water during an energetic workout.

Prawns bought with their shells on have a better flavour than those already shelled.

PRAWNS AND BULGUR WHEAT

225g/8oz/1 cup bulgur wheat
500ml/17fl oz/ 2 cups hot
   vegetable stock
1 red onion, finely diced
400g/14oz cooked and
   peeled prawns
2 handfuls basil, chopped

Place the bulgur wheat in a pan, pour over the stock and leave to stand for 30 minutes. Stir in the raw onion, prawns and basil, and serve.

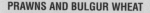

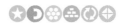

oyster

This delicious shellfish delicacy provides protein, B-vitamins and a massive dose of minerals.

The highest natural source of the mineral zinc, oysters are great for boosting immunity and improving the quality of sperm. A great source of energy for athletes, oysters are an excellent form of low-fat protein. They also contain vitamin B12, which helps to prevent pernicious anaemia, and iodine, vital for the proper functioning of the thyroid gland, which, if under-active, can lead to seriously debilitating bouts of exhaustion.

NUTRIENTS
Vitamins A, B3, B12, C, D, E; calcium, iodine, iron, magnesium, selenium, zinc; omega-3 essential fatty acids

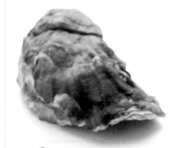

ROASTED OYSTERS

16 fresh oysters
1 tbsp sesame oil
1 tbsp white wine vinegar
1 tbsp lemon juice
1cm/½in piece root ginger,
    peeled and grated
1 tsp salt

Place the oysters deep-shell down on a roasting tray and roast in a pre-heated oven at 200°C/400°F/Gas mark 6 for 5 minutes until they open. Whisk the sesame oil, white wine vinegar, lemon juice, ginger and salt in a bowl. Flip off the top shells, and add a drizzle of dressing to each oyster. Serve the oysters in their shells as a starter.

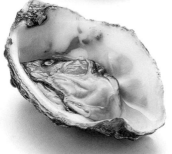

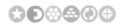

mussel

Crammed with joint-protecting essential fatty acids, muscles are a great food for anyone who regularly pounds the pavements.

NUTRIENTS
Vitamins B2, B6, B12, E, folic acid; calcium, iron, magnesium, potassium, selenium, zinc; omega-3 essential fatty acids

An average portion of mussels provides half a day's recommended intake of omega-3 fatty acids, which are great for their anti-inflammatory properties, helping to keep joints well oiled and preventing common sports injuries. Mussels are also exceptionally rich in zinc, a mineral essential for the breakdown of carbohydrates, fats and proteins into energy.

SEAFOOD SALAD

300g/10½oz cooked and
 shelled mussels
115g/4oz cooked and
 peeled prawns
1 onion, grated
½ white cabbage,
 shredded
2 carrots, peled and grated
1 beetroot, peeled and grated
2 tbsp mayonnaise

Combine the mussels, prawns, onion, white cabbage, carrots and beetroot in a large bowl. Mix in the mayonnaise well and serve.

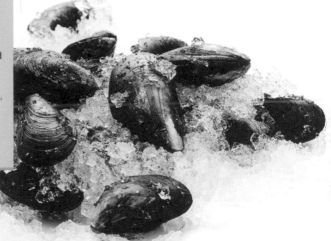

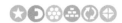

scallop

A type of mollusc with a soft, fleshy texture and a delicate, mild flavour, scallops are loaded with heart-friendly nutrients.

Scallops provide four nutrients that have significant cardio-vascular benefits for sportsmen and -women – vitamin B12, omega-3 essential fatty acids, magnesium and potassium. Vitamin B12 is needed by the body to counteract homocysteine, a chemical that can directly damage blood vessel walls; omega-3 fats help the blood to flow smoothly; magnesium encourages blood vessels to relax, lowering blood pressure; and potassium aids in the maintenance of normal blood pressure levels.

NUTRIENTS
Vitamin B12; calcium, magnesium, phosphorus, potassium, selenium; omega-3 essential fatty acids

GRILLED CORIANDER SCALLOPS

115g/4oz butter
juice of ½ lime
a small handful coriander
  leaves, chopped
24 scallops, shelled and
  shells reserved

Place the scallops flesh side up on a baking tray. Cook under a hot grill for 2 minutes. Divide the butter, lime juice and coriander between the shells. Cook for another 2–3 minutes until the scallops are white all the way through, and serve.

The edible part of the scallop is known as the "nut".

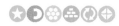

squid

NUTRIENTS

Vitamins B2, B3, B6, B12; calcium, iodine, magnesium, manganese, phosphorus, potassium, selenium, zinc; omega-3 essential fatty acids

With its distinctive, sweet taste, squid meat contains higher levels of immunity-boosting zinc, manganese and copper than many other seafoods.

Scientists have found that the proteins contained in squid meat are the same kinds of proteins found in fish meat, and are equal in nutritional value. With virtually no saturated fat, eight essential amino acids and a high level of easily digestible protein, squid is a good way for exercisers to get the increased protein they need to compensate for the increased muscle breakdown that occurs during and after intense exercise.

SALT AND PEPPER SQUID

1 tbsp salt
1 tbsp peppercorns
4 tbsp cornflour
4 tbsp semolina
800g/1lb 12oz squid, cleaned
1 litre/35fl oz/4 cups vegetable
  oil for deep frying
mayonnaise, to serve
lemon wedges, to serve

Crush the salt and pepper with a mortar and pestle, and mix with the cornflour and semolina in a bowl. Toss the squid in the mixture to coat. In a pan, fry ithe squid in hot oil until golden, then drain. Serve immediately with mayonnaise and lemon wedges.

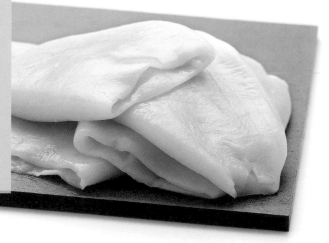

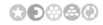

cod roe

Loaded with nutrients as well as tasting delicious, cod roe makes a fitness-friendly topping for toast.

NUTRIENTS
Vitamins A, B1, B2, B3, C, E; calcium, iron, magnesium; omega-3 essential fatty acids

Made up of the eggs of the female fish, cod roe is a wonderful source of vitamins D and E, containing almost as much vitamin E as an equivalent portion of wheat germ (the highest plant source of vitamin E). The omega-3 fatty acids provide all the raw materials the body needs to produce anti-inflammatory compounds that soothe post-workout aches and pains, and the protein slowly releases energy to drip-feed the muscles after an exercise session or sports match.

COD ROE ON TOAST

400g/14oz cod roe
3 tbsp plain flour
2 tbsp olive oil
a large handful
    rocket leaves
4 slices buttered
    wholemeal toast
juice of ½ lemon

Cut the cod roe into 1cm/½in slices. Lightly coat it in the flour and gently fry it in the oil for 3 minutes on each side. Arrange the rocket leaves on the toast, add the cod roe, drizzle over the lemon juice and serve.

A 175g/6oz portion of cod roe provides more than double the daily requirement of vitamin D.

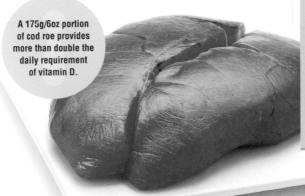

beef

NUTRIENTS
Vitamins B1, B2, B3, B6, B12; iron, phosphorus, selenium, sulphur, zinc; omega-3 essential fatty acids

An excellent source of protein and iron, beef helps anyone who's physically active to stay fighting fit.

The body's iron stores are depleted through perspiration, plus the impact of the feet hitting the ground when running destroys red blood cells, which means it's common for athletes to be deficient in this important mineral. Beef is a rich animal source of iron, which is easier to absorb than plant sources. It also contains conjugated linoleic acid, which stimulates the conversion of stored fat into energy.

HOME-MADE BEEF BURGERS

85g/3oz/½ cup long-grain rice
1 small onion
1 egg
a pinch salt
350g/12oz lean minced beef
1 tbsp olive oil

In a pan, cook the rice in 125ml/4fl oz/½ cup water. Blend the onion, egg and salt together in a food processor. In a bowl, mix the minced beef and cooled rice thoroughly with the egg mixture. Mould into burger shapes. Fry in the olive oil for 7 minutes on each side or until cooked as desired.

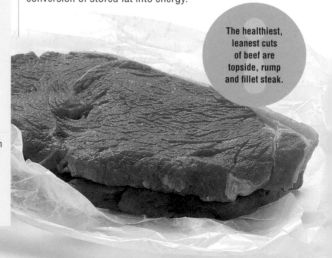

The healthiest, leanest cuts of beef are topside, rump and fillet steak.

lamb

Protein-rich lamb helps to prevent hunger pangs on the pitch or track, or in the studio or gym.

A lamb shank or loin is a lean cut of meat loaded with protein, which helps to suppress the appetite for longer and prolongs satiety more than foods high in carbohydrate or fat. Lamb is also rich in the mineral sulphur, a key component of chondroitin sulphate, a complex molecule that gives cartilage the elastic, sponge-like quality that joints need to act as shock absorbers between the bones.

NUTRIENTS
Vitamins B1, B2, B3, B6, B12; iron, phosphorus, selenium, sulphur, zinc

LAMB AND POTATO TRAYBAKE

800g/1lb 2oz new potatoes
8 bay leaves
2 red onions, sliced
2 tbsp olive oil
juice of 1 lemon
8 lamb loin chops
a handful mint, chopped

Put the potatoes, bay leaves and onions on a baking tray. Sprinkle with a little olive oil and the lemon juice, cover with foil and roast in a pre-heated oven at 220°C/425°F/Gas mark 7 for 40 minutes. In a pan, brown the chops on both sides in the remaining oil. Remove the foil, add the chops and mint, and roast for a further 15 minutes.

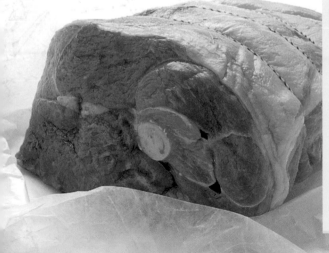

pork

NUTRIENTS
Vitamins B1, B2, B3, B6, B12; potassium, selenium, zinc

Pork is a valuable source of two trusty energy providers – protein and the B-vitamin complex.

While eating in general raises the metabolic rate, protein boosts it the most: up to 20 per cent of a protein meal's calories may be burned off. An average portion of pork (100g/3½oz) contains 30g/1oz of pure protein. It also has a full house of B-vitamins, which are essential for converting carbohydrates into energy and preventing fatigue.

ROAST GAMMON WITH PLUM GLAZE
serves 8

125g/4½oz plum jam
juice and zest of 1 orange
1 tsp ground nutmeg
1 tsp ground cinnamon
1 tsp ground ginger
2.25kg/5lb unsmoked
    gammon joint

Place the jam, orange and spices in a small pan, gently heat together and brush the mixture over the joint. Wrap joint in foil and roast in a pre-heated oven at 190°C/375°F/Gas mark 5 for 2½ hours. Remove the foil roast for a further 30 minutes. Carve and serve.

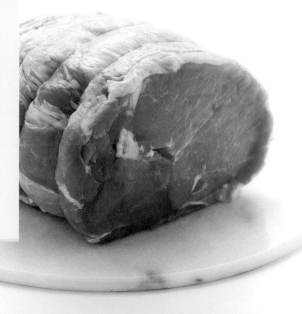

turkey

This low-fat, high-protein poultry has incredible muscle-building benefits.

NUTRIENTS
Vitamins B2, B3, B6, B12; iron, phosphorus, selenium, zinc

Scientists have found that turkey contains one of the highest concentrations of muscle-building substances called dipeptides. In tests, athletes who regularly ate 140g/5oz portions of turkey breast meat showed an increase of 40 per cent in muscle concentration, and performance improved greatly, especially for runners, rowers, cyclists and speed skaters.

Turkey leg meat contains twice as much iron and three times as much zinc as breast meat.

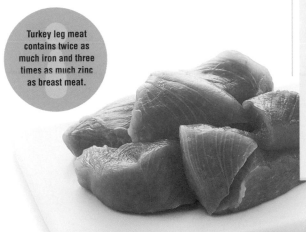

TURKEY SCHNITZEL

4 x 175g/6oz turkey breasts, flattened
3 tbsp plain flour
1 large egg, beaten
115g/4oz/4 cups cornflakes, finely crushed
green salad, to serve

Coat the turkey pieces lightly in the flour. Dip them in the egg and then coat in the cornflakes. Place on a baking tray and bake in a pre-heated oven at 180°C/350°F/Gas mark 4 for 25 minutes, until the juices run clear. Serve with a green salad.

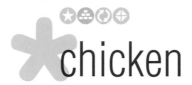

chicken

NUTRIENTS
Vitamins A, B2, B3, B6, B12, K; iron, magnesium, phosphorus, potassium, selenium, sodium, zinc

CHICKEN FACTS
*A chicken breast with the skin on contains almost twice as much saturated fat as a skinned chicken breast.

*The white breast meat of chicken contains less fat and fewer calories than the dark meat (wings and legs).

*Free-range poultry doesn't contain any of the growth-promoting hormones or antibiotics given to intensively reared birds.

*Chicken is cooked when it's opaque and there's no trace of pink at the bone, and the juices run clear.

Rated as a protein powerhouse, chicken is perhaps the most versatile meat of all.

A high intake of saturated fats increases the risk of heart disease and piles on the kilos/pounds, significantly slowing an athlete down. While all meat and dairy products contain some saturated fat, chicken, particularly if organic, is one of the leanest, most health-enhancing choices.

ENHANCES PERFORMANCE
Chicken provides a good deal of protein to build and repair muscles and an impressive list of minerals, including

---

BALSAMIC CHICKEN DRUMSTICKS

6 tbsp balsamic vinegar
2 tbsp sunflower oil
1 tsp Dijon mustard
1 tsp clear honey
½ tsp salt
1 tsp freshly ground
  black pepper
8 large chicken drumsticks

In a bowl, mix the vinegar, oil, mustard, honey, and season. Coat the drumsticks, and chill in a shallow dish for 2 hours. Grill for 15–20 minutes, turning every 5 minutes until cooked through and the juices run clear, then serve.

magnesium to help reduce the risk of cramps during exercise, and potassium to balance the fluid levels in the body, as well as selenium and zinc to bolster immunity. Zinc is also known to have energy-boosting properties.

LIFTS MOOD

Chicken is an excellent source of tryptophan, an essential amino acid that helps to control the brains serotonin levels, which are linked to appetite and mood. The B-complex vitamins also help to regulate the metabolism.

A 1–1.35kg/2–3lb chicken can be frozen whole for up to eight months and will take 10–12 hours to thaw.

THAI CHICKEN

1 tsp chilli powder
2.5cm/1in piece root ginger, peeled and grated
juice and zest of 1 lime
4 boneless chicken breasts, cut into strips
400ml/14fl oz/1½ cups coconut milk
400ml/14fl oz/1½ cups chicken stock

In a bowl, mix the chilli powder, ginger, and lime juice and zest. Place the chicken in a dish, pour over the marinade, cover and chill for 1 hour. Bring the remaining ingredients to the boil in a pan. Add the chicken and simmer for 15 minutes,.

duck

Eating roasted or stir-fried duck is an energy-rich way for athletes to hit their daily protein target.

Duck is a good source of protein and iron, both needed to repair tissue and build new cells. It is high in B-vitamins, which combat fatigue and regulate metabolism. Although duck has a reputation as a fat-laden meat, the saturated fat content is five times lower when all the skin is removed. In fact, a skinless duck breast is leaner than a skinless chicken breast.

NUTRIENTS
Vitamins B1, B2, B3, B6, B12; copper, iron, phosphorus, selenium, zinc

DUCK STIR-FRY

1 red onion, finely chopped
1 tbsp sesame oil
2 tbsp soy sauce
4 Mallard duck breasts, skinned and cut into strips
2 carrots, cut into batons
400g/14oz mung bean sprouts
juice and zest of 1 orange

Fry the onion in a wok in the oil and soy sauce. Add the duck breast strips and carrots and fry for 5 minutes. Then, add the bean sprouts and orange juice and zest, and cook for 1 further minute.

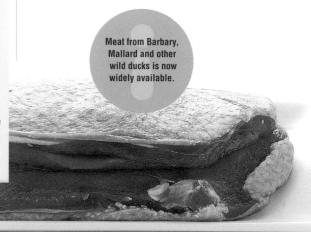

Meat from Barbary, Mallard and other wild ducks is now widely available.

054

rabbit

With its strong gamey flavour, rabbit helps to revive get-up-and-go.

Like other types of game, rabbits get plenty of exercise so their meat is leaner and lower in fat and calories than beef, lamb and pork, although equal in the protein stakes. Rabbit meat also contains iron and many of the B-vitamin complex, which all perform useful individual functions in the body, but work best together to ward off general tiredness and lethargy and thus boost energy levels for exercise.

NUTRIENTS
Vitamins B1, B2, B3, B6, B12; iron, phosphorus, zinc

RABBIT CASSEROLE

1 rabbit, skinned, boned
    and chopped into chunks
1 tbsp plain flour
1 tbsp vegetable oil
2 onions, chopped
a handful rosemary, chopped
125ml/4fl oz/½ cup
    chicken stock
125ml/4fl oz/½ cup dry
    white wine

Dip the rabbit chunks in the flour and lightly fry in the oil in an ovenproof dish. Add the remaining ingredients and bring to the boil. Cover and cook in a pre-heated oven at 180°C/350°F/Gas mark 4 for 2–2½ hours until tender.

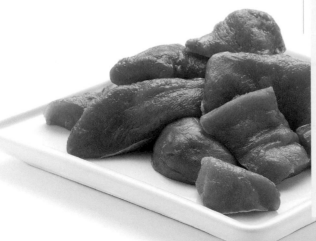

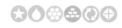

milk

NUTRIENTS
Vitamins A, B2, B12, D, E, K; calcium, iodine, phosphorus, potassium; omega-3 essential fatty acids

Known primarily as a bedtime sleep-inducer, a milky drink makes the perfect sports drink, too.

Milk contains many nutrients, including calcium to strengthen bones, vitamin E to boost immunity and potassium to protect the heart. Studies show that drinking chocolate milk improves endurance more than conventional carbohydrate-only sports drinks, because it contains the ideal ratio of carbohydrates to protein to help refuel tired muscles. Try a home-made milkshake, a smoothie or a cup of cocoa within two hours of exercise. The body converts these post-exercise calories into glycogen to deliver carbohydrate straight to fuel-depleted muscles.

> Organic milk contains 70 per cent more omega-3 fatty acids than non-organic milk.

BEDTIME MILK *serves 2*

500ml/17fl oz/2 cups milk
a tiny pinch saffron
2 tbsp clear honey
1 tsp grated nutmeg
½ tsp ground cinnamon

Gently heat the milk, saffron and honey in a pan, stirring until the honey is dissolved. Pour into cups, sprinkle over the spices and serve.

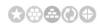

bio-yogurt

A brilliant bone-protector, bio-yogurt can be useful for sports players unable to tolerate lactose.

Bio-yogurt has a high calcium content, as well as traces of vitamin D, which help the body to absorb calcium and other bone-building minerals, such as magnesium and phosphorus. Eating it regularly reduces the risk of developing the bone-thinning condition, osteoporosis. Even people who can't digest dairy products because their body doesn't produce an enzyme called lactase, can usually eat yogurt – the live cultures in bio-yogurt produce their own lactase.

NUTRIENTS
Vitamins A, B2, B3, B5, B12, C, D, folic acid; calcium, iodine, iron, magnesium, phosphorus, potassium, selenium, zinc

HEALTHY COLESLAW

4 tbsp natural bio-yogurt
2 tsp Dijon mustard
2 tsp lemon juice
1 small white cabbage, shredded
4 carrots, peeled and grated
1 red onion, thinly sliced

Whisk together the yogurt, mustard and lemon juice in a bowl. Toss in the cabbage, carrots and red onion, mixing well. Serve as a side dish.

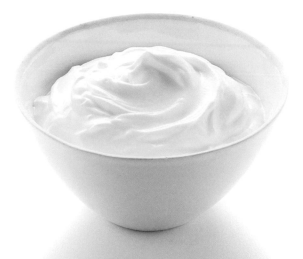

cheese

NUTRIENTS
Vitamins A, B2, B12; calcium, iodine, phosphorus, selenium

Eating cheese tops up the body's levels of calcium and protein – nutrients crucial for regular exercisers.

Weight-bearing exercise builds strong bones, but it puts them under pressure, increasing the body's need for calcium, which builds bone density. This means that cheese makes an ideal snack for athletes or sports players, who also lose calcium in perspiration. In fact, 30 minutes of sweat-inducing exercise increases calcium requirement. Cheese can get a bad press for its high saturated-fat content, but studies show that eating it after a meal actually boosts the body's ability to burn fat.

REALLY CHEESY SAUCE

55g/2oz butter
2 tbsp plain flour
400ml/14fl oz/1½ cups
    semi-skimmed milk
85g/3oz Stilton, crumbled
55g/2oz Parmesan, grated
½ tsp mustard
a pinch cayenne pepper
½ tsp grated nutmeg
wholemeal pasta, to serve

Melt the butter in a pan, add the flour and a little of the milk and stir to form a paste. Stirring over a gentle heat, add the rest of the milk. Bring to the boil, then remove from the heat. Add the Stilton and Parmesan, and stir in the mustard, cayenne pepper and nutmeg. Serve over wholemeal pasta.

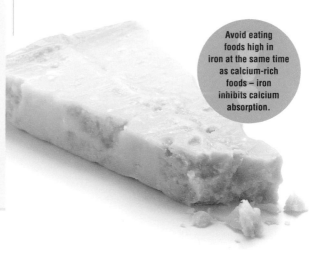

Avoid eating foods high in iron at the same time as calcium-rich foods – iron inhibits calcium absorption.

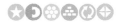

egg

The perfect complete protein, eggs contain all the essential amino acids needed by athletes.

Eggs are an excellent source of B-vitamins, zinc, iron and phospholipids – fats required for cell membranes and a healthy brain. They're also one of the few non-meat sources of vitamins A and B12, and D, which we need for healthy bones. Moreover, eggs are rich in vitamin K, which helps to heal bruises and other minor sports injuries by ensuring that blood is able to clot normally.

NUTRIENTS
Vitamins A, B2, B3, B5, B6, B12, D, E, folic acid; calcium, chromium, copper, iodine, iron, magnesium, manganese, phosphorus, potassium, selenium, sodium, zinc; omega-3 essential fatty acids

SMOKED SALMON OMELETTE

4 eggs
25g/1oz smoked salmon, chopped
1 tbsp olive oil
green salad, to serve

Beat the eggs and mix in the salmon. Heat the oil in a non-stick frying pan and pour in the egg mixture. Cook the omelette for 2 minutes until it is set at the edges, then use a spatula to flip the omelette and cook for 30 seconds on the other side. Serve with a green salad.

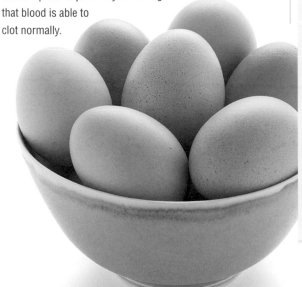

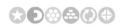

walnut

The only nut-source of omega-3 essential fatty acid, walnuts make an ideal daily snack for non-fish-eating athletes.

Like all nuts, walnuts are rich in anti-inflammatory, heart-healthy monounsaturated fats, which are important as a concentrated source of energy for anyone who's physically active. Unlike other nuts, walnuts also contain alpha-linoleic acid, an omega-3 essential fatty acid crucial for well-oiled joints and positive mood. Just 25g/1oz of walnuts a day provides half the adult daily quota of this important nutrient.

VEGETARIAN WALNUT BURGERS

175g/6oz/walnuts, shelled
4 slices wholemeal bread,
  toasted
1 red onion, coarsely chopped
2 eggs, beaten
55g/2oz Gorgonzola, crumbled
a handful chives

Grind the walnuts in a food processor. Add the toast, then the remaining ingredients and process to form a firm mixture. Shape into 1.5cm/½in patties. Bake in a pre-heated oven at 190°C/ 375°F/Gas mark 5 for 25–30 minutes until crisp, then serve.

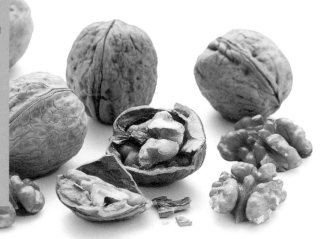

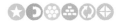

almond

Nibbling on almonds provides nutrients and energy for people who work out, with less risk of piling on unwanted pounds.

With more dietary fibre, calcium and vitamin E than any other nut, plus protein and heart-friendly monounsaturated fat, almonds are a nutritional powerhouse. It's thought that almonds help the body to burn fat more efficiently, as researchers found that of two groups of people on low-calorie diets, those who ate almonds daily lost 50 per cent more fat. This makes the nuts useful for anyone trying to shed fat and build muscle.

NUTRIENTS
Vitamins B1, B2, B3, B5, B6, E, folic acid; calcium, copper, iodine, iron, magnesium, manganese, phosphorus, potassium, selenium, zinc; omega-6 essential fatty acids

ALMOND MACAROONS
makes 20

2 large egg whites
175g/6oz/1¾ cups ground
    almonds
85g/3oz/⅓ cup caster sugar
1 tsp almond extract
a pinch salt

In a bowl, whisk he egg whites to form firm peaks. Fold in the almonds and sugar, then the almond extract and salt. Roll out and cut into 20 rounds. Place on a greased baking tray and bake in a pre-heated oven at 180°C/350°F/Gas mark 4 for 20 minutes until golden.

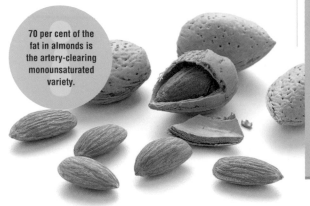

70 per cent of the fat in almonds is the artery-clearing monounsaturated variety.

✪⟐✳⟐⟐⊕

hazelnut

NUTRIENTS
Vitamins B1, B3, B6, E, folic acid; iron, calcium, magnesium, manganese, potassium; omega-9 essential fatty acids

A popular ingredient in rich chocolates, hazelnuts also make a scrumptious and nutritious snack in their own right.

Containing plenty of fibre, vitamins, minerals and protein, raw hazelnuts are a nutrient-dense snack choice. They are particularly rich in omega-9 fatty acid, a monounsaturated fat also known as oleic acid, which boosts the immune system. This helps the body to ward off performance-impairing coughs and colds, and is especially important for anyone who regularly trains outdoors near pollution-causing traffic.

HAZELNUT SHORTBREAD

115g/4oz butter
85g/3oz/⅓ cup caster sugar
1 egg, beaten
2 tsp instant coffee, dissolved in 2 tbsp boiling water
200g/7oz/1⅔ cups plain flour
55g/2oz/½ cup ground hazelnuts
55g/2oz/½ cup ground almonds

In a bowl, beat the butter and sugar until creamy, then fold in the egg and coffee. Stir in the flour and nuts to form a dough. In between 2 sheets of baking paper, roll out to a thickness of 1cm/½in and refrigerate overnight. Cut into squares and bake on a tray in a pre-heated oven at 150°C/300°F/Gas mark 2 for 25 minutes until golden.

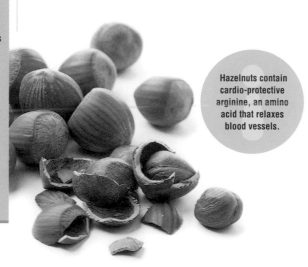

Hazelnuts contain cardio-protective arginine, an amino acid that relaxes blood vessels.

062

pine nut

Pine nuts are perfect with pasta, in stir-fries or salads, or as an energy-boosting snack.

The small edible seeds of the pine tree, pine nuts are lower in fat content than most other nuts, which means they're a brilliant choice for weight-conscious athletes who need to get plenty of muscle-building protein and joint-friendly essential fats in their diet without overloading on calories. High in immunity-boosting antioxidant vitamin E, pine nuts are also nature's only source of pinoleic acid, a substance found to stimulate the hormones that help to diminish appetite.

NUTRIENTS
Vitamins D1, B2, B3, E; copper, iron, magnesium, manganese, zinc; omega-6 essential fatty acids

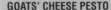

GOATS' CHEESE PESTO

115g/4oz/¾ cup pine nuts
115g/4oz soft goats' cheese
25g/1oz Parmesan, grated
55g/2oz basil leaves
55g/2oz sun-dried tomatoes
juice of 1 lemon
2 garlic cloves, crushed
a pinch cayenne pepper

Place all the ingredients in a food processor and blend until smooth.

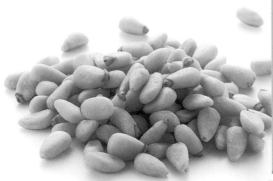

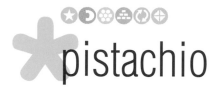

pistachio

These easy-to-open, pale green nuts are heart-smart and help to maintain good eyesight.

NUTRIENTS
Vitamins B1, B3, E; calcium, copper, magnesium, manganese, potassium, zinc; omega-6 essential fatty acids

Cardiovascular fitness is central to any exercise regime and studies show that eating 25g/1oz of monounsaturated fat-loaded pistachio nuts a day decreases the incidence of heart disease between 20 and 60 per cent.

STRENGTHENS BONES

PISTACHIO FACTS
*The pistachio nut is a member of the cashew family.

*Pistachio trees are planted in orchards, and take up to ten years to produce a significant amount of nuts.

*One serving of pistachio nuts (about 45 kernels) provides as much potassium as half a banana.

*Pistachio nuts contain seven amino acids.

Pistachios are a good choice because they're also packed with the minerals essential for optimum fitness. Calcium keeps the bones strong; copper increases energy, protects joints and helps the body to utilize iron; magnesium combats muscle fatigue; and zinc speeds up recovery from muscular injuries.

PISTACHIO AND MANGO LASSI *serves 1*

½ mango, peeled and chopped
3 tbsp natural bio-yogurt
55g/2oz pistachios, shelled
2 tsp caster sugar

Blend the mango, yogurt, nuts, sugar and 125ml/4½fl oz/½ cup water in a food processor. Serve over ice.

PROTECTS EYESIGHT

Pistachios are also the only nuts that contain high levels of lutein and zeaxanthin, antioxidants needed to maintain eye health, which is particularly important in racquet and team sports where good hand–eye and foot–eye co-ordination is a key skill.

PISTACHIO COUSCOUS

250g/9oz/1 cup couscous
4 cardamom pods, crushed
1 tsp salt
a handful mint
115g/4oz pistachios, shelled
½ tsp grated nutmeg

Bring 500ml/17fl oz/2 cups water to the boil in a pan. Reduce the heat, add the couscous, cardamom, salt and mint, and simmer for 10 minutes. Remove from the heat, fork through the nuts, add the nutmeg and serve.

Pistachio nuts are known as the "smiling nut" in Iran and the "happy nut" in China.

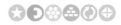

cashew

Cashew nuts make a handy, nutrient-loaded snack when you've worked up an appetite exercising.

Cashew nuts are rich in many of the minerals that active people need. For example, 30 cashews provide one-fifth of a woman's recommended daily iron intake, while 20 nuts provide more than one-tenth of a man's daily zinc requirement. The phosphorus in the nuts works with the calcium to form and maintain strong bones, while the copper has healing properties, and may help to rid the body of infections.

CASHEW NUT DIP

115g/4oz/⅓ cup cashew nuts
1 tbsp crunchy peanut butter
3 garlic cloves, crushed
3 tbsp olive oil
juice of 1 lemon
100g/3½oz/⅓ cup tahini
a pinch paprika
pitta bread, to serve

Blend all the ingredients in a food processor until smooth. Serve with pitta bread.

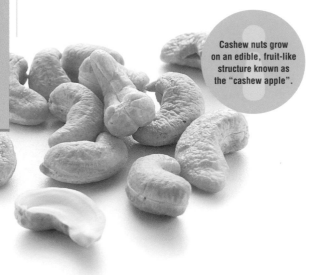

Cashew nuts grow on an edible, fruit-like structure known as the "cashew apple".

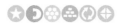

Brazil nut

These mineral-rich marvels are great for perking up anyone whose fitness levels are flagging.

Brazil nuts are renowned for their high selenium content, a nutrient with potent antioxidant properties, which reduces the risk of heart disease and cancer. Selenium also lifts a low mood, helping to relieve depression, anxiety and fatigue. Four Brazil nuts provide the recommended daily amount of selenium. Brazils are also rich in magnesium, which is important for the formation of protein and boosting energy levels.

NUTRIENTS
Vitamins B1, E; calcium, copper, iron, magnesium, manganese, phosphorus, selenium, zinc; omega-3 and -6 essential fatty acids

CHOCOLATE-DIPPED BRAZILS

55g/2oz dark chocolate
1 tbsp crystallized ginger, finely chopped
100g/3½oz Brazil nuts, shelled

Break the chocolate into pieces, and melt in a heatproof bowl over a pan of simmering water. Stir in the ginger and coat the nuts in the mixture. Place on a baking tray lined with greaseproof paper, ensuring that they don't touch. Refrigerate them until the chocolate hardens.

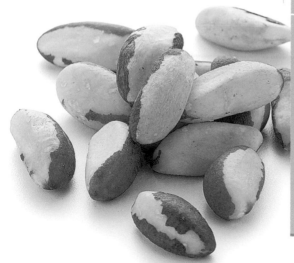

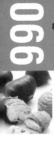

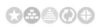

chestnut

NUTRIENTS
Vitamins B1, B2, B6, C, folic acid; potassium

Chestnuts have the lowest fat and the highest carbohydrate content of all nuts, as well as a pleasantly sweet flavour.

The low-fat, high-carbohydrate content of chestnuts is a dream combination for anyone watching their calorie intake and wishing to boost their energy levels before a work-out. Unlike other tree nuts, the insides of chestnuts are not hard, but soft and fleshy, and cannot be eaten raw as they contain very high levels of tannic acids, which can cause digestive discomfort. This means they need to be boiled or roasted before eating.

CHESTNUT AND BUTTER BEAN SOUP

400g/14oz/3 cups chestnuts, cooked and peeled
400g/14oz/2 cups tinned butter beans
3 shallots, chopped
1 carrot, peeled and chopped
1 parsnip, peeled and chopped
500ml/17fl oz/2 cups stock

Place all the ingredients in a pan, cover and bring to the boil. Reduce the heat and simmer for 20 minutes. Purée until smooth.

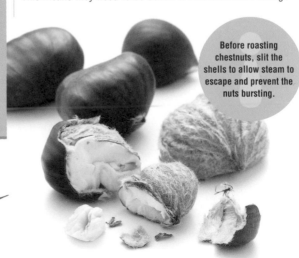

Before roasting chestnuts, slit the shells to allow steam to escape and prevent the nuts bursting.

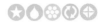

coconut

Easily digested and metabolized by the body, coconut is a great pre-exercise energy source.

Although coconut is high in saturated fats known as medium-chain fatty acids (MCFAs), these don't pose the same negative health risk as other saturated fats. This is because the body uses them as instant energy rather than storing them as fat. The coconut water – the liquid inside the coconut – is known to be one of the most balanced natural electrolyte sources, making it a wonderfully rehydrating drink after intensive exercise.

NUTRIENTS
Vitamins B1, B2, B3, B5, B6, C, E, folic acid; calcium, copper, iodine, iron, magnesium, manganese, phosphorus, potassium, selenium, zinc

COCONUT RICE

225g/8oz/1 cup brown rice
1 onion, chopped
1 tbsp ground coriander
1 tbsp ground cumin
2 tbsp coconut oil
2 beef tomatoes, chopped
3 tbsp desiccated coconut

Place the rice and 500ml/ 17fl oz/2 cups water in a pan and bring to the boil. Reduce the heat and simmer for 45 minutes. In another pan, fry the onion and spices in the oil for 3 minutes. Add the tomato and coconut, and simmer for 10 minutes. Mix well with the rice. Serve as a side dish.

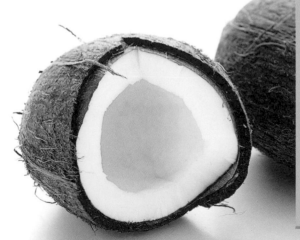

✪ ☽ ✣ ✤ ✪ ✤

pumpkin seed

NUTRIENTS
Vitamins B2, B3, B5, E, K,
beta-carotene; calcium, copper,
iron, magnesium, manganese,
phosphorus, potassium, zinc;
omega-3 and -6 essential
fatty acids

Boasting the highest iron content in the seed world,
pumpkin seeds make a very nutritious nibble.

The easily absorbed iron in pumpkin seeds encourages the
formation of red blood cells and helps to ensure that oxygen
is pumped around the body efficiently, making fatigue and low
energy levels during exercise less likely. These seeds are rich
in omega-3 oils, which are anti-inflammatory and protect joints
from damage during high-impact activities. They also promote
the healing of sports-related injuries.

PUMPKIN-SEED GRANOLA

2 tbsp maple syrup
100g/3½oz/1 cup rolled oats
2 tbsp coconut oil
4 tbsp pumpkin seeds
1 tbsp sesame seeds
2 tbsp ground almonds
1 tbsp desiccated coconut

In a pan, fry the syrup and oats
in the oil over a low heat for 3
minutes. Mix in the seeds,
almonds and coconut. Spread
on a baking tray and bake at
150°C/300°F/Gas mark 2 for
25 minutes. Allow to cool,
then serve.

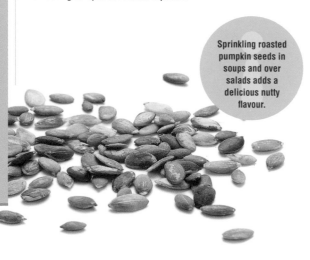

Sprinkling roasted
pumpkin seeds in
soups and over
salads adds a
delicious nutty
flavour.

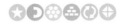

flaxseed

Thanks to their essential fatty acids, flaxseeds are hailed as "superseeds" across the globe.

Flaxseeds are top of the nutrition league when it comes to heart-healthy and joint-friendly omega-3 content. They provide calcium for bone strength and magnesium to help ward off muscle cramps and release energy. As flaxseeds and their oils are easily oxidized, which causes them to go rancid, keep them in dark bottles or tubs with sealed lids, and store them in the fridge for no longer than a year.

NUTRIENTS
Calcium, magnesium, zinc; omega-3 essential fatty acids

FLAXSEED MUFFINS
makes 12

115g/4oz/½ cup golden flaxseeds, ground
175g/6oz/1¼ cups wholemeal flour
1 tbsp baking powder
2 tsp ground allspice
200g/7oz/1 cup brown sugar
1 egg, beaten
250ml/9fl oz/1 cup milk

Mix the dry ingredients in a bowl. Add the egg and milk. Spoon into 12 muffin cases in a muffin tin and bake in a pre-heated oven at 180°C/350°F/Gas mark 4 for 25 minutes.

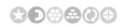

sesame seed

NUTRIENTS

Vitamins B1, B2, B3, B5, B6, E, beta-carotene; calcium, copper, iodine, iron, magnesium, manganese, phosphorus, potassium, zinc; omega-6 essential fatty acids

A fantastic source of calcium, sesame seeds are brilliant non-dairy bone-builders.

These tiny seeds are often used to make tahini or sesame paste, or simply scattered over stir-fries, salads and pasta. They are packed with calcium, containing more of this important mineral than most foods, including whole milk. Sesame seeds are also a great source of vitamin-B complex, which, together with the omega-6 essential fatty acids, help to keep the heart healthy and release energy to enhance stamina and fight fatigue.

NUTTY BANANA PUDDING

**175g/6oz/heaped 1 cup
  roasted peanuts
55g/2oz/½ cup butter
2 tbsp maple syrup
1 tbsp tahini
4 whole bananas, peeled
55g/2oz/⅓ cup
  sesame seeds**

Grind the peanuts in a blender. In a pan, gently melt the butter and stir in the syrup, tahini and ground peanuts. Coat each banana evenly with the peanut mixture, then sprinkle the sesame seeds over them. Allow to cool and serve.

In ancient India, sesame seeds were a symbol of immortality.

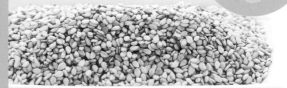

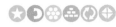

sunflower seed

Eating sunflower seeds helps to maintain a healthy heart, which is key to reaching optimum fitness.

Sunflower seeds are an excellent source of vitamin E, the body's primary fat-soluble antioxidant, whch does the important job of neutralizing harmful free radicals, promoting healthy blood flow and regulating the heartbeat. These seeds also contain lots of magnesium, crucial for healthy bones and muscles. Other potent minerals found in sunflower seeds include selenium and zinc, which protect from disease.

NUTRIENTS
Vitamins B1, B2, B5, E, folic acid; calcium, copper, iron, magnesium, manganese, phosphorus, selenium, zinc; omega-6 essential fatty acids

TABBOULEH WITH SUNFLOWER SEEDS

200g/7oz/1 cup bulgur wheat
400ml/14fl oz/1½ cups hot
   vegetable stock
4 tbsp sunflower seeds
2 tbsp flaxseeds
1 red onion, coarsely chopped
½ cucumber, diced
a handful parsley, chopped
a handful mint leaves,
   chopped

In a bowl, mix the bulgur wheat and stock, cover and leave for 30 minutes. Fork through the remaining ingredients and serve.

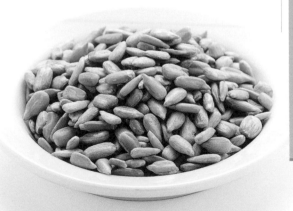

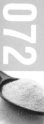

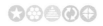

corn

NUTRIENTS
Vitamins B3, B5, C, folic acid;
calcium, magnesium,
potassium, zinc

Cornmeal and cornflour are nutritious gluten-free options for anyone who can't tolerate wheat.

Ground into meal or flour, corn is a useful kitchen-cupboard staple for making bread and tortillas and for thickening sauces and puddings. It's a complex carbohydrate, which means it keeps blood sugar stable for longer during exercise. Also, research has found that switching from white flour to lower-fat whole-grain corn helps to prevent anaemia, because it increases the absorption of iron by up to 50 per cent.

CORN CRISPBREAD

85g/3oz/⅔ cup cornflour
150g/5oz/ heaped 1 cup
brown rice flour
4 tbsp milk
½ tsp salt

In a bowl, mix all the ingredients to make a soft dough. On a floured surface, roll out to a thickness of 5mm/¼in and cut into rectangles. Place on a greased baking tray and bake in a pre-heated oven at 200°C/400°F/Gas mark 6 for 8–10 minutes until golden.

Yellow cornmeal
is also known
as maize
and polenta.

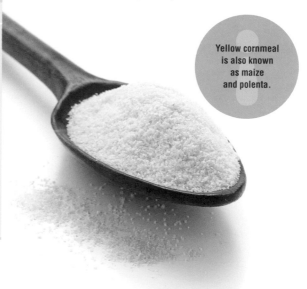

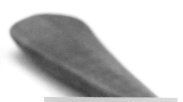

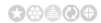

barley

Barley is the perfect pre-race fuel-provider for long-distance runners, cyclists and swimmers.

This glutinous grain has a chewy texture similar to pasta and is an excellent source of complex carbohydrate, which means it balances blood-sugar levels and releases energy slowly over time to give endurance athletes more strength and stamina. It's also a great source of B-vitamins, which also help to boost energy. All types of barley are nutrient-rich, but pot barley retains much more fibre than pearl barley. Soak barley overnight in cold water before adding to warming soups or stews.

NUTRIENTS
Vitamins B1, B2, B3, B5, B6, B9, B12, folic acid; calcium, iron, magnesium, manganese, phosphorus, potassium, selenium, zinc

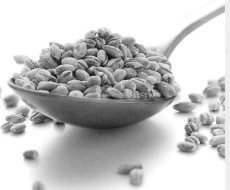

BAKED BARLEY

125g/4½oz/⅔ cup pearl barley
1 onion, finely chopped
1 tbsp olive oil
1 tbsp tomato purée
a handful basil, chopped
a handful thyme
juice of ½ lemon

Bring 400ml/13fl oz/1⅔ cups water to the boil in a heatproof casserole dish. Stir in all the ingredients, cover and bake in a pre-heated oven at 190°C/375°F/Gas mark 5 for 30–40 minutes. Fluff with a fork and serve.

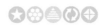

millet

NUTRIENTS
Vitamins B1, B2, B3, B5, B6, E,
K, folic acid; calcium, copper,
iron, magnesium, manganese,
phosphorus, potassium, selenium,
silica, zinc

This king of the complex carbohydrates helps to keep the body strong for optimum fitness.

Easy to digest, millet is high in silica, needed for healthy tendons and bones. This small, round grain is also protein-rich, containing all the eight essential amino acids that aid recovery from sports-related injuries. Unlike most grains, millet is alkaline-forming, so it may help to neutralize acidic conditions that affect the joints, such as arthritis. It's also high in B-vitamins, which are known to boost energy and combat stress. Millet is loaded with the health-enhancing minerals calcium and magnesium, which are essential for building strong bones.

MILLET PORRIDGE

250ml/9fl oz/1 cup
  semi-skimmed milk
115g/4oz/½ cup millet
55g/2oz raisins
2 tsp clear honey
a pinch nutmeg

Pour the milk and 125ml/
4fl oz/½ cup water into a pan
and add the millet. Bring to
the boil, reduce the heat and
simmer for 15 minutes. Stir in
the raisins and honey. Sprinkle
over the nutmeg and serve.

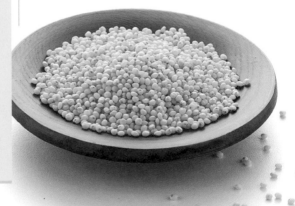

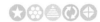

rye

A high-fibre low-GI grain, rye makes a great pre-workout snack, as it staves off hunger pangs and helps to prevent fluid retention.

With more insoluble fibre and less gluten than wheat, rye is a wholegrain cereal that's commonly milled into flour and made into stamina-building bread. This is ideal for athletes, as it releases energy slowly, preventing hunger pangs and energy dips. Rye is rich in plant lignans, which help to reduce blood viscosity, and sucrose and fructooligosaccharide, which have prebiotic properties that help to prevent bloating.

NUTRIENTS
Vitamins B1, B2, B3, B5, B6, B9, B12, E; calcium, iron, magnesium, manganese, phosphorus, potassium, selenium, zinc

RYE BREAD

100g/3½oz/1 cup dark rye flour
350g/12oz/2¾ cups plain flour
10g/¼oz dried active yeast
50g/1¾oz/¼ cup soft dark brown sugar
2 tsp salt
1 egg, beaten
1 tbsp vegetable oil

Mix the flours, yeast, sugar and salt in a bowl. Mix in the egg, oil and 250ml/9fl oz/1 cup warm water and knead for 10 minutes. Cover the dough and leave for 1 hour until doubled in size. Knead into a ball and leave on an oiled baking tray for 30 minutes. Bake in a pre-heated oven at 200°C/400°F/Gas mark 6 for 30–35 minutes.

Rye bread, such as pumpernickel, is widely eaten across Central and Eastern Europe.

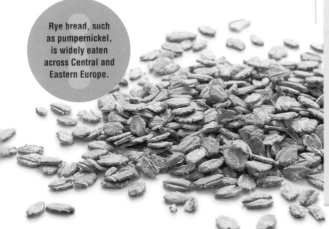

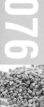

buckwheat

NUTRIENTS
Vitamins B1, B2, B3, B5, B6, E, K, folic acid; calcium, copper, iron, magnesium, manganese, phosphorus, potassium, selenium, zinc

Eating this wholesome grain can reduce the risk of broken veins and chilblains while training outdoors in winter.

Buckwheat is extremely rich in a natural chemical called rutin, which keeps the inner lining of blood vessels clear and helps to prevent chilblains and broken veins. For anyone with a wheat or gluten allergy, soba noodles, which can be found in supermarkets, are often made with 100 per cent gluten-free buckwheat. These noodles have an earthy, grain-like taste and can be used hot or cold in salads and stir-fries.

BUCKWHEAT BLINIS
makes 12–14

250ml/9fl oz/1 cup milk
1 egg
1 tsp olive oil, plus extra
for frying
55g/2oz/½ cup buckwheat flour
55g/2oz/⅓ cup wholemeal flour
a pinch salt

In a food processor, blend the milk, egg and oil together. Add the flours and salt, and blend until smooth. Heat a little oil in a non-stick pan and fry a tablespoon of batter to make each blini, cooking for 2 minutes on each side.

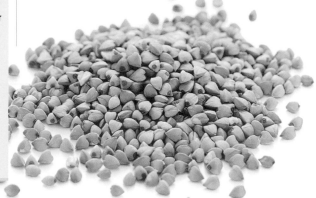

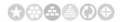

amaranth

This tiny, nutritious wholegrain is a fantastic source of complete protein and complex carbohydrates.

Researchers found that athletes who ate a low-GI wholegrain, such as amaranth, before exercise were able to keep going considerably longer than those who ate a high-GI, white-flour-based food. It's also been found that low-GI grains can help the body to burn more fat during exercise. Amaranth contains more iron and calcium than most other grains, helping to boost overall energy levels and bone strength.

NUTRIENTS
Vitamins B1, B2, B3, B5, B6, C, E, folic acid; calcium, copper, iron, magnesium, phosphorus, potassium, zinc

AMARANTH PUDDING

125g/4½oz/1¼ cups amaranth
250ml/9fl oz/1 cup milk
55g/2oz/½ cup ground almonds
55g/2oz/¼ cup caster sugar
1 tbsp cocoa powder
55g/2oz dark chocolate

Mix the amaranth, milk, almonds, sugar and cocoa in a large pan, cover and bring to the boil. Reduce the heat and simmer for 15 minutes. Pour into four bowls, grate over the chocolate and serve.

Amaranth was a staple grain for the Aztec civilization of central Mexico.

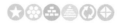

oats

NUTRIENTS
Vitamins B1, B2, B3, B5, B6, E, K, folic acid; calcium, copper, iron, magnesium, manganese, phosphorus, potassium, selenium, silica, zinc

Usually eaten as energy-packed porridge and in flapjacks and cereal bars, oats regularly feature in line-ups of the "top ten" superfoods.

Oats release their energy very slowly and can keep an athlete going for hours, because they are an excellent source of wholegrain complex carbohydrates. They also contain more protein than most other grains and are bursting with soluble fibre, which helps to eliminate cholesterol from the body. Whole oats (also known as groats) consist of the whole grain with the hull removed. Rolled oats are whole oats that have been flattened between rollers.

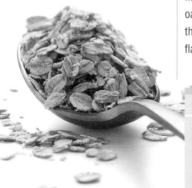

OATY BREAKFAST PANCAKES *makes 10–12*

2 large eggs	Blend the eggs, butter, sugar and cinnamon in a food processor. Stir in the oats and baking powder. In a pan, fry tablespoons of the batter in the oil, cooking on each side for 1–2 minutes.
55g/2oz butter	
1 tbsp soft brown sugar	
1 tsp ground cinnamon	
125g/4½oz/1¼ cups rolled oats	
1 tbsp baking powder	
1 tbsp vegetable oil	

wheat

Wheat often gets a bad press, but it can be a top source of carbohydrate for endurance athletes.

NUTRIENTS
Vitamins B1, B2, B3, E, folic acid; copper, iron, magnesium, manganese, phosphorus, zinc

A reduction in the body's carbohydrate stores is one of the major causes of fatigue during prolonged exercise. White flour doesn't provide many nutrients, but other wheat sources are a nutritious way to top up carbohydrate levels. Have wholegrain pasta as a pre-exercise meal, beef up a smoothie with wheatgerm (the tiny seed found inside the wheat grain) or use bulgur wheat (a mineral-rich cracked wheat grain) in place of white rice.

Wheat is the world's most widely cultivated plant, grown on every continent except Antarctica.

CREAMY GREEN SPAGHETTI

300g/10½oz wholemeal
  spaghetti
55g/2oz/⅔ cup coarse fresh
  wholemeal breadcrumbs
zest of 1 lime
1 garlic clove, crushed
225g/8oz watercresss
250ml/9fl oz/1 cup
  single cream
½ tsp grated nutmeg

In a pan, cook the spaghetti in boiling salted water for 12 minutes. Drain and cover. In a bowl, mix the breadcrumbs with the lime zest and garlic, spread on a baking tray and grill for 3–4 minutes. Drain the spaghetti and stir in the breadcrumbs, watercress and cream. Sprinkle over the nutmeg and serve.

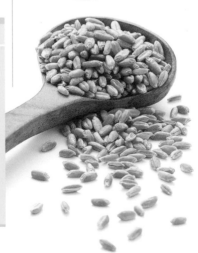

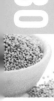

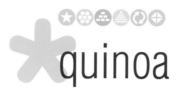

quinoa

Vitamins B1, B2, B3, B5, B6,
E, folic acid; calcium, copper,
iron, magnesium, manganese,
phosphorus, potassium, zinc

Pronounced "keen-waa", quinoa is one of the best sources of protein in the plant kingdom.

Strictly speaking, quinoa is a seed, not a grain. Low in fat, it's full of slow-release carbohydrates, which balance the blood sugar.

BUILDS STRENGTH

Containing all eight essential amino acids, quinoa is an exceptionally rich source of protein, making it a useful addition

Quinoa is loaded with lysine, an amino acid that is essential for tissue growth and repair.

QUINOA-STUFFED PEPPERS

250g/9oz/½ cup quinoa
1 onion, chopped
2 garlic cloves, crushed
115g/4oz mushrooms,
  chopped into
  small pieces
1 tbsp olive oil
4 red peppers

In a pan, bring 500ml/17fl oz/ 2 cups water to the boil. Add the quinoa, reduce the heat and simmer for 15 minutes. In another pan, soften the onion, garlic and mushrooms in the oil. Add the quinoa and mix well. Cut the tops off the peppers and remove the cores and seeds. Fill each pepper with the mixture, replace the tops and place in an ovenproof dish. Bake in a pre-heated oven at 190°C/375°F/Gas mark 5 for 45 minutes.

to the diet of regular exercisers and serious athletes, who need more protein than inactive people. (An insufficient intake delays the body's recovery after training and slows the development of muscle and stamina.)

BOOSTS ENERGYY

A serving of quinoa provides nearly the entire spectrum of B-vitamins, needed to boost energy and combat stress, as well as lots of vitamin E, a key component in skin health and the body's healing process. Quinoa is also rich in calcium and magnesium, essential for healthy bones, iron to help prevent fatigue, and zinc to enhance the immune system.

QUINOA FACTS

*Quinoa was once called "the gold of the Incas", who recognized its value in increasing the stamina of their warriors.

*When quinoa is cooked, the grains become translucent and the white germ partially detaches itself, appearing like a white-spiralled tail.

*For a nuttier flavour, dry roast quinoa before cooking in a heavy-based pan over a medium-low heat, stirring constantly for 5 minutes.

*The leaves of the quinoa plant are edible, with a taste similar to its green-leafed relatives, spinach and chard.

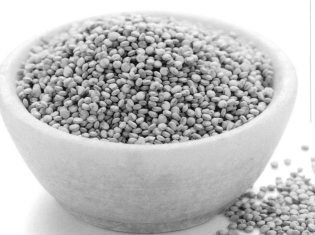

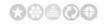

spelt

Containing more nutrients than its well-known distant cousin, wheat, this ancient grain is now regaining popularity.

NUTRIENTS
Vitamins A, B1, B2, B3, B6, E, folic acid; calcium, copper, magnesium, manganese, phosphorus, potassium, selenium, zinc

Used to make bread and pasta, spelt is exceptionally high in manganese. In fact, a 115g/4oz serving provides two-thirds of the recommended daily intake of this trace mineral, which is invaluable for athletes as it is vital for many bodily functions, including bone and connective tissue formation, thyroid function, calcium absorption, blood-sugar regulation and fat and carbohydrate metabolism. Spelt is also an important source of zinc and selenium, which boost immunity.

SPELT CRACKERS WITH TRICOLORE SALAD

2 avocados, peeled and pitted
juice of ½ lemon
8 spelt crackers
4 tomatoes, thinly sliced
115g/4oz mozzarella cheese, finely sliced
salt
freshly ground black pepper

In a bowl, mash the avocados with the lemon juice and season. Spread over the crackers, and top with a layer of tomato and mozzarella slices, then serve.

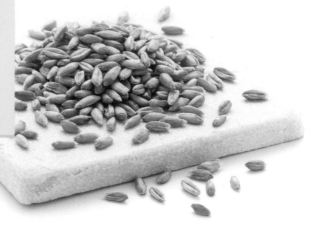

triticale

A nutritious alternative to wheat, triticale is a great source of carbohydrate, boosting stamina during matches and workouts.

NUTRIENTS
Vitamins B1, folic acid; calcium, iron, magnesium

Triticale is a hybrid of wheat and rye that was first bred in Sweden and Scotland in the late nineteenth century. Today, cracked triticale can be used in the same way as cracked wheat, and triticale flakes make a great substitute for oat flakes. It is high in folic acid, which protects against heart disease, as well as calcium and magnesium, crucial for healthy bones.

The word "triticale" is an amalgamation of the Latin words *triticum* (wheat) and *secale* (rye).

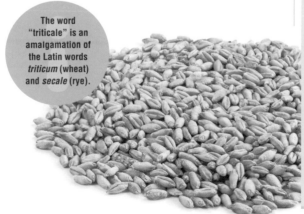

MUSHROOM BAKE

1 onion, finely chopped
500g/1lb 2oz mushrooms, halved
1 tbsp olive oil
100g/3½oz/heaped ¾ cup triticale flour
1 tbsp tomato purée
a handful oregano

In a pan, fry the onion and mushrooms in the oil. In a bowl, mix the flour and tomato purée with 4 tablespoons water to form a paste. Add the oregano and mix all the ingredients together. Transfer to an oven-proof dish and bake in a pre-heated oven at 170°C/325°F/Gas mark 3 for 20 minutes.

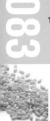

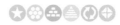

brown rice

NUTRIENTS
Vitamins B1, B3, B5, B6, E, K,
folic acid; calcium, copper, iodine,
iron, magnesium, manganese,
phosphorus, potassium,
selenium, zinc

With its nutty flavour, brown rice is a heart-warming grain that tastes good hot or cold.

Rice is one of the most easily digested grains, which is why rice cereal is often recommended as a baby's first solid. Retaining both the bran and germ of the rice kernel, brown rice is a source of protein, carbohydrates and fibre. Brown basmati rice contains more amylose than other types of rice, which means it is less rapidly absorbed into the body, providing a steady stream of energy for exercisers, rather than a spike followed by a slump.

INDIAN WHOLEGRAIN PILAFF

2 shallots, finely chopped
1 tsp ground cumin
1 tsp ground turmeric
1 tsp ground coriander
4 cloves
6 cardamom pods, crushed
15g/½oz butter
450g/1lb/2¼ cups brown rice

In a pan, fry the shallots
and spices in the butter for
3 minutes. Stir in the rice
for 2 minutes, add 900ml/
31fl oz/3¾ cups water. Bring
to the boil, reduce the heat
and simmer, covered, for
25 minutes.

Studies show that the oil in whole brown rice lowers blood cholesterol levels.

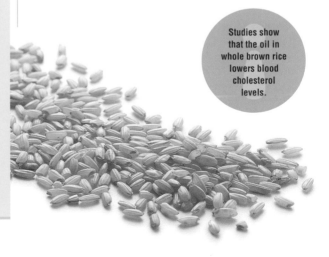

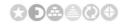

wild rice

Chewy in texture, wild rice is rich in protein, packed with dietary fibre and low in fat.

NUTRIENTS
Vitamins B1, B2, B3, E; iodine, phosphorus, potassium, selenium, zinc; omega-3 and -6 essential fatty acids

Wild rice is not really rice, but a type of grass containing twice the protein of white rice and fewer calories and fat. Nutritionally, it is one of the few grains that also provide the essential fatty acids omega-3 and -6, which are mostly found in oily fish, nuts and seeds. It's also an ideal pre-workout food, as it's an excellent source of the energy-boosting B-vitamins, thiamine (B1), riboflavin (B2) and niacin (B3).

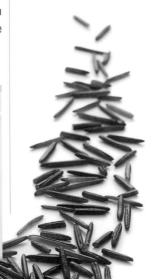

SALMON AND WILD RICE STEW

2 red onions, finely chopped
1 tbsp olive oil
100g/3½oz/½ cup wild rice
750ml/26fl oz/3 cups fish stock
100g/3½oz/½ cup basmati rice
500g/1lb 2oz salmon fillets,
  cut into large pieces
a handful dill, chopped
2 tbsp crème fraîche

In a pan, fry the onions in the oil until soft. Stir in the wild rice and stock. Bring to the boil and cook for 15 minutes. Add the basmati rice, cover, reduce the heat and cook for 20 minutes. Add the salmon. Cook for 7 minutes. Flake the salmon, then add the dill and crème fraîche.

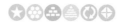

lentil

NUTRIENTS

Vitamins B3, B5, B6, B9, folic acid; calcium, iron, magnesium, manganese, phosphorus, potassium, selenium, zinc

SWEET AND SOUR LENTILS

250g/9oz/1 cup red lentils
2 tbsp vegetable oil
2 dried red chillies, chopped
½ tsp mustard seeds
2 tbsp soy sauce
1 tbsp sugar
4 tbsp pineapple juice
1 tbsp white wine vinegar

Place the lentils in a pan, cover with water and bring to the boil. Cover the pan, reduce the heat and simmer for 40 minutes; drain. In another pan, heat the oil and spices for 3 minutes. Add the soy sauce, sugar, juice, vinegar and lentils. Stir in 125ml/4fl oz/½ cup water, simmer for 10 minutes, then serve.

One of the best foods for endurance sports, lentils also provide a dose of the feel-good factor.

Packed with protein and slow-releasing natural sugars, lentils are great for stabilizing blood-sugar levels and maintaining stamina. In fact, one study found that eating lentils three hours before exercise could help to increase endurance significantly more than other carbohydrates. Lentils are also crammed full of folic acid, an energy-boosting vitamin that plays a key role in the production of serotonin, the neurotransmitter in the brain associated with feeling happy.

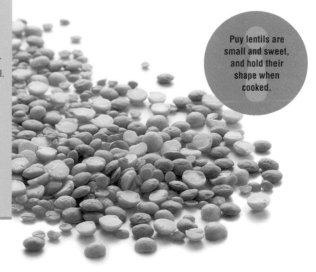

Puy lentils are small and sweet, and hold their shape when cooked.

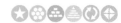

chickpea

Chickpeas are handy hormone balancers for female athletes prone to performance-impairing PMS.

Throughout the Middle East, India and Latin America, chickpeas are a stomach-filling staple. Rich in plant hormones known as isoflavones, which mimic oestrogen in the body, chickpeas can help to prevent hormone-related conditions, such as PMS and menopausal hot flushes. Thanks to their high B-vitamin content, chickpeas also support the functions of nerves and muscles, while their high carbohydrate content provides energy.

NUTRIENTS

Vitamins B1, B2, B3, B5, B6, E, K, beta-carotene, folic acid; calcium, copper, iodine, iron, magnesium, manganese, phosphorus, potassium, selenium, zinc

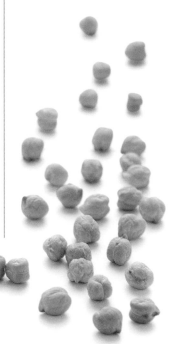

CHICKPEA SALAD

225g/8oz/1½ cups dried
  chickpeas
10 spring onions, thinly sliced
200g/7oz watercress
200g/7oz rocket leaves
a handful mint
3 tbsp olive oil
2 tbsp balsamic vinegar
115g/4oz Parmesan shavings

Soak the chickpeas overnight. Drain, place in a pan and cover with water. Bring to the boil, reduce the heat and simmer for 2 hours until soft. Once cool, mix well with the onions, watercress, rocket, mint, oil and vinegar in a large bowl. Scatter over the cheese and serve.

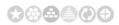

aduki bean

NUTRIENTS

Vitamins B1, B3, B5, B6, E, beta-carotene, folic acid; calcium, copper, iodine, iron, magnesium, manganese, phosphorus, potassium, selenium, zinc

Reduce pace-slowing water retention by including this tasty little pulse on the menu.

Containing more fibre and protein and less fat than most other beans, aduki beans are rich in B-vitamins for steady energy production and body tissue repair. They're also high in many minerals needed for optimal fitness: fatigue-fighting iron; potassium, which acts as a natural diuretic by helping the body to eliminate excess fluid; and immunity-boosting minerals zinc, calcium and magnesium.

ADUKI BEAN HOT POT

100g/3½oz/½ cup dried
    aduki beans
1 large onion, chopped
3 carrots, peeled and diced
2 parsnips peeled and diced
2 sweet potatoes, peeled
    and diced
2 bay leaves
1 tbsp tomato purée

Soak the beans overnight in cold water. Drain, put in a pan and cover with water. Bring to the boil, reduce the heat and simmer for 45 minutes. Drain. Put all the ingredients into a large casserole dish with water to cover. Bake in a pre-heated oven at 190°C/375°F/Gas mark 5 for 1½ hours.

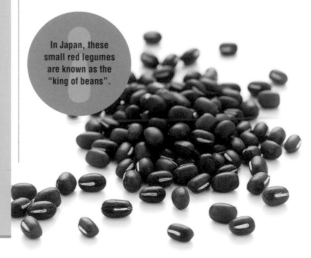

In Japan, these small red legumes are known as the "king of beans".

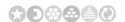

edamame

Snacking on edamame, loaded with protein, iron, carbohydrates and fibre, provides athletes with a serious stamina boost.

Edamame, which look like a cross between broad beans and peas, are baby soya beans prepared in the pod. Hailed as the latest superfood, the pods are picked while still young and tender. Very popular in Japan, China and Korea, edamame are high in fibre, bone-friendly protein and slow-releasing carbohydrates to help prevent mood fluctuations by keeping blood-sugar levels steady.

NUTRIENTS
Vitamins A, C, folic acid; calcium, iron; omega-3 essential fatty acids

ROASTED EDAMAME BEANS

1 tsp chilli powder
¼ tsp ground cumin
¼ tsp ground coriander
¼ tsp ground ginger
¼ tsp ground turmeric
a pinch paprika
2 tsp sunflower oil
400g/14oz/2 cups ready-to-eat
    edamame pods

In a small bowl, mix the spices with the oil. Toss the beans in the mixture and place on a baking tray. Bake in a preheated oven at 190°C/375°F/ Gas mark 5 for 10–15 minutes. Allow to cool. Serve as a snack.

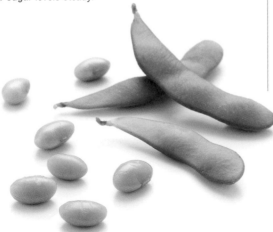

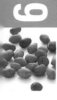

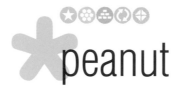

peanut

NUTRIENTS
Vitamins B3, E, folic acid; calcium, copper, magnesium, manganese, phosphorus, potassium

PEANUT FACTS
*Researchers have found that roasting peanuts can increase the level of a compound called p-coumaric acid, increasing their overall antioxidant content by up to 22 per cent.

*The potassium in peanuts helps to regulate the body's water levels and the normal metabolism of food, which prevents cramping, especially during a workout.

*To retain the optimal health benefits, opt for peanut butter made from peanuts only, with no added sodium, sugar or hydrogenated oil.

*Peanuts are one of the foods most commonly associated with allergic reactions.

Peanuts and peanut butter are packed with protein and heart-healthy fats – a great source of energy for exercise and sports.

In spite of their name, peanuts aren't a nut, but a legume. They're loaded with protein (20–30 per cent) to help muscles stay strong and have a low GI, which means they help to keep blood-sugar levels stable.

LOWER CHOLESTEROL
On the heart-health front, peanuts contain vitamin E, the amino acid arginine and oleic acid (the monounsaturated fat found in olive oil), all of which have been shown to reduce

---

PEANUT SQUARES

200g/7oz/1¼ cups roasted peanuts
1 tbsp chunky peanut butter
100g/3½oz/½ cup golden granulated sugar
1 tsp bicarbonate of soda
1 tsp cornflour

Finely grind the peanuts in a blender. In a large bowl, mix all the ingredients. Press into a small, greased baking tray. Bake at 160°C/325°F/Gas mark 3 for 25 minutes. Cool, cut into squares and serve.

high cholesterol levels in the blood and to protect against the formation of plaque in the arteries, which clogs them up.

FIGHT DISEASE
Peanuts also contain 30 times more resveratrol than grapes – resveratrol is one of a class of compounds called phytoalexins, associated with reduced cardiovascular disease.

Peanuts grow underground, which is why they're often referred to as groundnuts.

INDONESIAN-STYLE PEANUT SAUCE

115g/4oz/⅔ cup
  peanuts
juice and zest of 1 lime
250ml/9fl oz/1 cup
  coconut milk
1 tbsp tamarind paste
1 tbsp curry powder
6 spring onions,
  finely chopped
chicken, to serve

Blend the peanuts and lime juice and zest in a blender to form a paste. Transfer to a pan and stir in the remaining ingredients and 125ml/4fl oz/ ½ cup water. Cook over a gentle heat for 7 minutes. Serve over chicken.

butter bean

NUTRIENTS
Vitamins B1, B3, B5, folic acid;
copper, iron, magnesium,
manganese, molybdenum,
phosphorus, potassium, zinc

BUTTER BEAN AND BROCCOLI SOUP

2 onions, chopped
2 tsp grated nutmeg
2 tbsp olive oil
1.5 litres/52fl oz/6 cups
  vegetable stock
450g/1lb/2½ cups tinned
  butter beans, drained
450g/1lb broccoli florets
1 large potato, peeled and
  chopped into 2.5cm/1in cubes

Gently cook the onions and
nutmeg in a pan in the oil for
5 minutes. Add the stock,
beans, broccoli and potato.
Bring to the boil, reduce
the heat and simmer for
15 minutes until tender.
Purée in a blender and serve.

This soft, floury bean has lots of digestion-friendly fibre and powerful detoxifying properties.

Like all beans, butter beans are loaded with fibre, and can be a good source of protein, vital to athletes for bone strength when combined with other vegetable proteins, such as rice or quinoa. Butter beans are especially rich in the trace mineral, molybdenum, which has been shown to help the body detoxify toxic sulphites – a type of preservative linked to headaches and asthma-like symptoms, which is added to processed foods, "deli" salads, baked goods and wine.

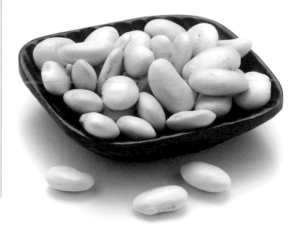

kidney bean

A Mexican food staple, these versatile beans work well in chillis, salads, dips and wraps.

One average serving of kidney beans provides lots of protein and one third of the recommended daily intake of fibre. This is beneficial for regular exercisers who want to lose weight, because fibre curbs hunger for longer, while the protein gives energy. Kidney beans are also rich in folic acid, which helps to speed up wound healing – useful for anyone prone to blisters.

NUTRIENTS
Vitamins B1, B6, K, folic acid; copper, iron, magnesium, manganese, molybdenum, phosphorus, potassium, zinc

MEXICAN BEAN DIP

250g/9oz/1½ cups dried
  kidney beans
½ onion, finely chopped
½ tsp chilli powder
1 tbsp olive oil
2 tbsp sour cream
2 tbsp chopped
  coriander

Soak the kidney beans in cold water overnight. Drain, put in a pan and cover with water. Boil for 10 minutes, reduce the heat, simmer for 2 hours and mash. In another pan, fry the onion and chilli powder in the oil for 5 minutes. Allow to cool, then purée with the kidney beans, sour cream and coriander in a blender, and serve.

Kidney beans are highly toxic if consumed raw, so always eat cooked or tinned beans.

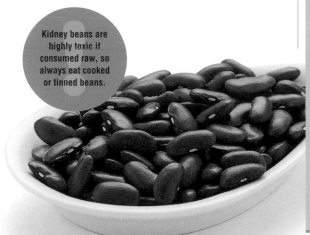

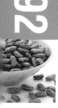

pinto bean

NUTRIENTS
Vitamin B1, B6, folic acid; copper, iron, magnesium, manganese, phosphorus, potassium, selenium, zinc

Stay "full of beans" with this excellent low-fat, low-calorie source of protein.

Combine the creamy pink texture of pinto beans with a whole grain such as brown rice for a virtually fat-free, high-quality protein meal. Pinto beans are especially rich in the amino acid lysine, which is lacking in most other plant proteins. One serving provides around a quarter of the recommended daily intake of iron, which is essential for transporting oxygen around the body and keeping up energy levels during exercise.

PINTO BEAN FUDGE

175g/6oz dark chocolate
  (70 per cent cocoa)
85g/3oz butter
4 tbsp semi-skimmed milk
85g/3oz/1 cup drained,
  tinned pinto beans,
  mashed
1 tsp peppermint extract
900g/2lb/7¼ cups icing sugar

In a small pan, gently melt the chocolate and the butter, then add the milk. Add the pinto beans and peppermint extract, then gradually add the sugar, stirring to form a thick mixture. Spread the mixture over a greased baking tray, then cover and refrigerate. Once set, chop into squares and serve.

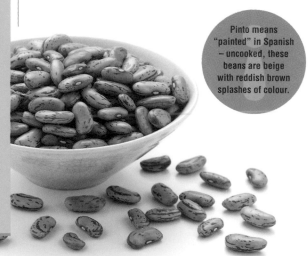

Pinto means "painted" in Spanish – uncooked, these beans are beige with reddish brown splashes of colour.

093

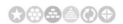

soya bean

Soya beans contain more protein than dairy products and have similar bone-protecting properties.

The top-ranking pulse on the nutritional scale, soya beans are a source of complete protein, as they contain all eight amino acids. Soya beans are loaded with isoflavones, hormone-like plant chemicals particularly helpful for female athletes, as they help to balance oestrogen levels in the body and protect against osteoporosis by increasing bone mass. Soya beans also contain B-vitamins, which play a role in helping the body to cope with stress.

NUTRIENTS
Vitamins B1, B2, B3, B5, B6, E, K, beta-carotene, folic acid; calcium, copper, iodine, iron, magnesium, manganese, phosphorus, potassium, selenium, zinc

BANANA, AVOCADO AND SOYA SMOOTHIE
serves 2

1 ripe banana, peeled
1 avocado, peeled and pitted
100g/3½oz silken tofu
400ml/14fl oz/1½ cups
  soya milk
a generous sprinkling
  flaked almonds

Whizz together the banana, avocado, tofu and soya milk in a blender until smooth. Sprinkle over the flaked almonds and serve immediately.

garlic

Acclaimed as a wonderfood, garlic guarantees extra protection for overworked joints and helps to keep the heart healthy, too.

Exercise places increased strain on the joints and can sometimes set up an inflammatory response in the body. Consuming a clove of garlic a day has been proven to counteract inflammation. A sulphur compound in garlic known as allicin has been found to aid weight loss and to protect against heart disease by preventing fatty deposits forming inside the arteries. Its selenium and zinc content also boost immunity.

GARLIC MUSHROOM SALAD

4 garlic cloves, crushed
12 large open mushrooms
3 tbsp olive oil
4 handfuls rocket leaves
115g/4oz feta cheese

In a pan, gently fry the garlic and mushrooms in the oil. Arrange the rocket leaves in four piles on four plates. Put three mushrooms on each pile, crumble over the cheese, and serve.

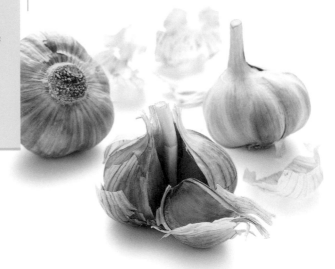

ginger

With its great pain-relieving and circulation-boosting properties, ginger is a useful addition to any athlete's diet.

Ginger is useful for anyone feeling sluggish because it is stimulating and promotes detoxification by increasing perspiration and circulation. Recognized by scientists as a fast-acting cure for nausea of all kinds, fresh ginger also contains anti-inflammatory compounds called gingerols, which suppress the substances that trigger joint pain and swelling. In addition, ginger is particularly rich in the mineral zinc – essential for a healthy immune system.

NUTRIENTS
Vitamin B3, B6, C, E, folic acid; calcium, copper, iron, magnesium, manganese, phosphorus, potassium, selenium, zinc

GINGERADE
serves 2

1 tbsp caster sugar
55g/2oz fresh root ginger, peeled and grated
250ml/9fl oz/1 cup sparkling mineral water
juice of ½ lemon

Place the sugar, ginger and 250ml/9fl oz/1 cup water in a pan and bring to the boil. Reduce the heat, cover and simmer for 10 minutes. Leave to cool and pass through a sieve. Stir into the sparkling mineral water, add the lemon juice and serve with ice.

For a post-match or post-race reviver, pour hot water on grated ginger and drink as a tea.

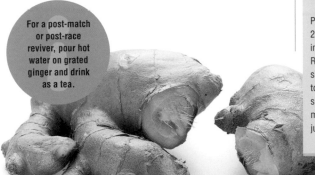

960

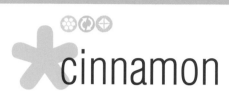

cinnamon

NUTRIENTS
Vitamins B2, B3, B5, B6, E, K, beta-carotene; calcium, copper, iodine, iron, magnesium, manganese, phosphorus, potassium, selenium, zinc

CINNAMON FACTS
*Cinnamon is a spice made from the inner bark of the *Cinnamomum zeylanicum* tree. The bark is stripped from the tree and allowed to dry in the sun. While drying, it rolls up into a quill (sold as a cinnamon stick). Some of the quills are then ground into a powder.

*Cinnamon is one of the oldest-known spices. It was mentioned in ancient Chinese writings 2,700 years ago and features several times in the Bible.

*Ceylon cinnamon has a lighter, sweeter and more delicate flavour than the Indonesian variety.

This fragrant spice provides a satisfying alternative for athletes who find it difficult to resist unhealthy sugary snacks.

STABILIZES BLOOD SUGAR
Research has shown that compounds in cinnamon stabilize blood-sugar levels, which in turn prevent mood swings and dips in blood sugar post-exercise – a time when even the most health-conscious athlete might be tempted to succumb to calorie-laden chocolate and sweets. As little as half a teaspoonful a day – sprinkled on porridge for breakfast or used to sweeten a cup of herbal tea – can make a difference and, say scientists, even help to control type-2 diabetes.

APPLE AND CINNAMON PORRIDGE

2 cinnamon sticks	In a large pan, bring 750ml/
5 cloves	26 fl oz/3 cups of water to the
2 tsp sugar	boil. Reduce the heat, add the
2 apples, peeled	cinnamon, cloves, sugar
and sliced	and apple, and simmer for
125g/4½oz/1¼ cups	10 minutes. Remove the spices,
instant porridge oats	stir in the oats and serve.

PREVENTS THRUSH

Cinnamon also has anti-bacterial and anti-fungal propertles that have been found to inhibit organisms such as *Candida albicans*, a yeast responsible for causing candidiasis and thrush.

Cinnamon's distinct smell works directly on the brain to increase alertness.

CINNAMON TEA

4 heaped tsp black tea leaves
4 cinnamon sticks
1 lemon, sliced

Place the black tea, cinnamon sticks and lemon slices in a pan and pour over 1 litre/35fl oz/ 4 cups freshly boiled water. Allow to steep for 5 minutes. Pour through a strainer into four cups and serve.

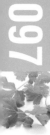

parsley

Vitamins A, B1, B3, B5, C, E, K, folic acid; calcium, copper, iodine, iron, magnesium, manganese, phosphorus, potassium, selenium, zinc

One of the world's most popular culinary herbs, parsley helps to balance fluid levels in the body, especially important after a hard training session.

The richest herbal source of the mineral potassium, parsley is a natural diuretic, encouraging the excretion of sodium and water. This helps to balance fluid levels in the body, which can be disturbed by exercise. Curly English and broadleaf Continental parsley are both excellent sources of the fatigue-fighting duo, iron and vitamin C. Both have been used traditionally to improve arthritic conditions.

PARSLEY SAUCE

25g/1oz butter
1 tbsp plain flour
400ml/14fl oz/1½ cups milk
2 tbsp double cream
juice and zest of
  ½ lemon
4 tbsp parsley, finely
  chopped
freshly ground black pepper

In a small pan, gently melt the butter, then stir in the flour to form a smooth paste. Gradually add the milk, bring to the boil, and reduce the heat. Simmer for 3 minutes, whisking constantly. Add the cream, lemon juice and zest and parsley, and season with black pepper.

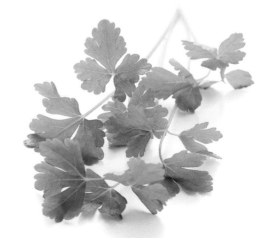

860

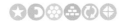

tofu

One of the best vegetarian forms of protein for athletes, tofu works well in everything from smoothies to stir-fries.

NUTRIENTS
Vitamins A, K; calcium, copper, iron, magnesium, manganese, phosphorus, potassium, selenium; omega-3 and -6 essential fatty acids

Aso known as bean curd, tofu is a versatile, low-fat food jam-packed with nutrients. Like all soya products, it is rich in phytoestrogens that help to regulate hormone levels, and calcium to build strong bones. Tofu is a good source of omega-3 fatty acids and fibre, which both help to stave off food cravings. It also contains an isoflavone called genistein, which seems to promote fat loss by reducing the size and number of fat cells.

> Soft tofu blends easily in smoothies and desserts; firm tofu works well in main meals.

BLUEBERRY AND TOFU MOUSSE

200g/7oz silken tofu
250g/9oz/1⅔ cups blueberries
85g/3oz/¾ cup ground almonds
1 tsp ground cinnamon
1 tsp lemon juice
2 tsp toasted, flaked almonds

Blend the tofu and blueberries in a food processor. Add the ground almonds, cinnamon and lemon juice. Spoon the mousse into four bowls and sprinkle over the almond flakes.

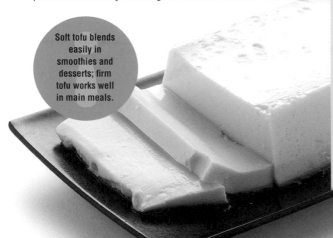

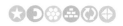

miso

NUTRIENTS
Vitamins B1, B2, B3, B5, B6,
K, beta-carotene, folic acid;
calcium, copper, iron, magnesium,
manganese, phosphorus,
potassium, selenium, sodium, zinc

Miso does more than just add flavour to soups and stews, it notches up their nutrient rankings, too.

A naturally fermented paste, miso is made from soya beans, sea salt and a yeast mould called *koji*. A handy store-cupboard staple, it is ideal for spicing up soups, sauces and stews. Miso is an excellent source of protein, and boasts a host of minerals to enhance an athlete's performance, including manganese, which strengthens nerves, bones and muscles, and phosphorus, necessary for the metabolism of fats, protein and glucose.

Dark miso contains more protein and essential fatty acids than lighter varieties.

MISO SANDWICH SPREAD

1 tbsp miso
1 tbsp tahini
1 garlic clove, crushed

Mix all the ingredients together well in a small bowl. Use over warm crusty wholemeal bread or use as a tasty substitute for butter in sandwiches.

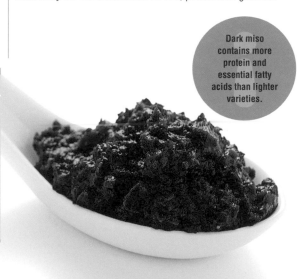

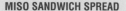

balsamic vinegar

Thanks to its alkalizing effect, balsamic vinegar is a useful ingredient for fitness lovers who are prone to muscle cramps.

Originally from the Modena province of Italy, this dark brown syrupy vinegar is made from reduced grape juice aged in wooden casks. Like all vinegars, balsamic is bursting with enzymes and trace minerals that help to balance the body's acid–alkaline levels. It is especially rich in the disease-fighting phytochemicals found in grapes, which become even more potent during the vinegar's fermentation process.

NUTRIENTS
Vitamins B1, B2, B6, C, E, beta-carotene; calcium, iron, magnesium, manganese, phosphorus, potassium, selenium, silica, sulphur, zinc

TANGY SALAD DRESSING

4 tbsp balsamic vinegar
juice and zest of 1 orange
juice and zest of 1 lime
1 tsp mustard
1 tbsp olive oil
2 garlic cloves, crushed

Place all the ingredients in a screw-top jar and shake well to combine. Store in the fridge for up to one week.

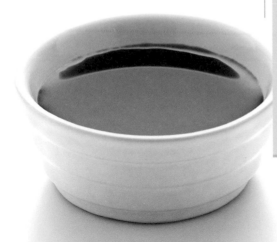

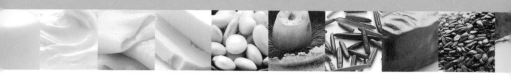

ailments directory

ANAEMIA

This condition occurs when there is a decrease in the amount of oxygen-carrying haemoglobin in our red blood cells. Symptoms include feeling tired all the time, weakness, pale skin, breathlessness and pale inner lower eyelids. Eating foods rich in iron and vitamin B12 can help to combat anaemia.

Foods to eat:

Plum (p.12); Broccoli (p.37); Chard (p.39); Beef (p.62); Lamb (p.63); Amaranth (p.93); Quinoa (p.96); Lentil (p.102)

ATHLETE'S FOOT

Athlete's foot is a common fungal infection characterized by itchy dry patches of skin between the toes that sometimes split open. It's highly contagious, often thriving on the damp floors of changing rooms and communal showers. Help your body to fight it off by avoiding refined sugar products and by limiting your consumption of yeast products, such as bread, alcohol and yeast extract.

Foods to eat:

Aubergine (p.46); Bio-yogurt (p.71); Garlic (p.112); Ginger (p.113); Cinnamon (p.114); Balsamic vinegar (p.119)

BLISTERS

A common sports ailment, blisters often form on the feet and heels. They are caused by friction on the outer layers of skin, forming fluid-filled sacks to protect the inner layers of skin from more damage. To prevent them, wear well-fitting trainers and socks. To help heal them, eat foods rich in vitamins C and K, which both speed up the healing process.

Foods to eat:

Star fruit (p.16); Goji berry (p.24); Chard (p.39); Pak choi (p.40); Eggs (p.73); Oats (p.94)

CRAMP

Cramp is the sudden uncontrolled contraction of a muscle, often in the thigh or calf. The exact cause is unknown, but it's thought that

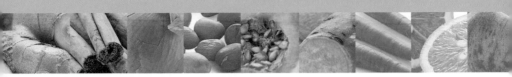

overexertion from exercise, muscle fatigue and excessive sweating (which depletes the body of minerals, such as sodium, potassium, magnesium and calcium) can all play a part. Anyone prone to regular cramps is wise to eat foods loaded with these important minerals.

Foods to eat:

Pear (p.10); Date (p.19); Papaya (p.21); Butternut squash (p.34); Prawn (p.56); Chicken (p.66); Cashew (p.80); Aduki bean (p.104)

DEHYDRATION

During exercise, the body loses fluids through perspiration. The amount depends on how hard and long you train, as well as the surrounding temperature and humidity. Losing the equivalent of two per cent of your body weight in sweat results in a 10–20 per cent drop in performance (or aerobic capacity). Severe dehydration can lead to vomiting and heat exhaustion. That's why it's recommended that athletes drink enough fluids every day to ensure they need to urinate every two to four hours so that the urine is lightly coloured and copious. The American College of Sports Medicine recommends drinking 150–350ml/5–12 fl oz water every 15–30 minutes during a workout. And an athlete should drink at least 2 litres/70fl oz/8 cups of liquid during the course of a day. You can also improve your hydration by eating foods with a high water content.

Foods to eat:

Plum (p.12); Peach (p.13); Lemon (p.14); Orange (p.15); Mango (p.20); Lychee (p.23); Milk (p.70); Coconut (p.83)

DEPRESSION (MILD)

Characterized by tearfulness, anxiety and feelings of hopelessness, mild depression is a condition experienced by one in four people at some stage in their lives. Cutting out alcohol, cigarettes and sugary foods and eating those high in omega-3 fatty acids and B-vitamins is thought to help. Exercise is also known to increase the feel-good factor.

Foods to eat:

Salmon (p.50); Tuna (p.51); Mackerel (p.53); Walnut (p.74); Quinoa (p.96); Spelt (p.98); Brown rice (p.100)

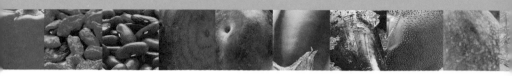

HEART DISEASE

One of the main causes of heart disease is the blockage of arteries by cholesterol. Following an exercise regime and eating monounsaturated fats (found in olive oil, nuts, seeds and fish) instead of saturated fats (found in animal products and processed foods) can make a dramatic difference to your heart health.

Foods to eat:

Avocado (p.25); Olive (p.26); Salmon (p.50); Tuna (p.51); Mackerel (p.53); Pistachio (p.78); Sunflower seed (p.87); Peanut (p.106)

HIGH BLOOD PRESSURE

Hypertension, or high blood pressure, means that the heart has to work harder to pump blood around the body, and increases the risk of heart disease and strokes. You can bring it down through exercise, stress reduction and losing excess weight. It also helps if you avoid high-fat and salt-laden dishes and opt instead for foods loaded with magnesium, vitamin C, essential fatty acids and fibre.

Foods to eat:

Orange (p.15); Goji berry (p.24); Broccoli (p.37); Mushroom (p.41); Trout (p.49); Oats (p.94); Lentil (p.102); Edamame (p.105)

INSOMNIA

An inability to drop off to sleep or a pattern of waking up during the night can lead to health problems such as fatigue, irritability and lower levels of concentration. Studies show that exercise and physical activity increase our mental alertness for four hours afterwards, so avoiding evening work-outs can help to prevent insomnia. Stimulants, such as coffee and chocolate, can also interrupt sleep patterns if you consume them less than five hours before bed. Instead, encourage sleep with foods rich in B-vitamins, magnesium, calcium and the amino acid, tryptophan.

Foods to eat:

Banana (p.11); Fig (p.18); Date (p.19); Chard (p.39); Sardine (p.52); Turkey (p.65); Milk (p.70); Egg (p.73)

JOINT PROBLEMS

Regular exercise can place a strain on the joints. For example, knee pain is a

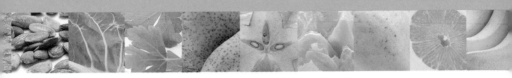

common running injury. It's possible to protect joints from injury and wear and tear by maintaining the correct weight for your height and by alternating periods of heavy activity with periods of rest to avoid repetitive stress on your joints. Research also shows that eating foods rich in essential fatty acids can help to protect the cartilage cells that facilitate joint movement.

Foods to eat:
Olive (p.26); Salmon (p.50); Mackerel (p.53); Walnut (p.74); Flaxseed (p.85); Wild rice (p.101); Garlic (p.112); Ginger (p.113)

OBESITY

You are described as being obese if your body weight reaches 20 per cent above the recommended maximum for your height. An exercise programme coupled with a nutrient-dense diet is key to shedding the extra weight.

Foods to eat:
Lettuce (p.28); Pepper (p.29); Bio-yogurt (p.71); Almond (p.75); Pine nut (p.77); Kidney bean (p.109); Tofu (p.117)

OSTEOPOROSIS

Osteoporosis causes bones to become weak so that you are more prone to fractures and breaks. Eating foods rich in calcium, as well as phosphorus and magnesium, can help to prevent the disease. Making sure you spend plenty of time outside also helps, as the sun triggers the production of vitamin D, which helps to turn the calcium you eat into bone.

Foods to eat:
Fig (p.18); Onion (p.31); Sardine (p.52); Milk (p.70); Bio-yogurt (p.71); Cheese (p.72); Sesame seed (p.86); Tofu (p.117)

POST-VIRAL FATIGUE (M.E.)

Although the specific cause of post-viral fatigue is still unknown, it often follows on from a viral illness and is more likely to occur in athletes who over-train. This chronic condition is characterized by low energy levels and poor concentration. Eating plenty of immunity-boosting fruit and vegetables can help to alleviate the symptoms.

Foods to eat:
Star fruit (p.16); Guava (p.22); Goji berry (p.24); Pepper (p.29); Beetroot (p.30); Carrot (p.33); Garlic (p.112)

glossary

Adrenaline A hormone released in response to stress that boosts the supply of oxygen and glucose to the brain and muscles.

Allicin A compound in garlic that has potent anti-bacterial and anti-fungal activities.

Amino acids Compounds, either made by the body or found in the diet, which are involved in processes such as the formation of neurotransmitters in the brain.

Anti-bacterial A substance that destroys or inhibits the growth of bacteria.

Anti-fungal A substance that destroys or inhibits the growth of fungi.

Anti-inflammatory A substance that prevents or reduces inflammation.

Antioxidants Compounds in fruit and vegetables that fight free radicals, preventing cell degeneration and decay.

Arginine An organic compound found in animal proteins.

Beta-carotene A fat-soluble vitamin found as carotenoids in plant foods, which the body converts into vitamin A.

Betaine A phytonutrient used by the liver to produce choline, a compound that promotes muscle growth.

Blood sugar The form in which fuel from food is carried in the blood to provide energy to cells.

Calorie A measurement of the energy the body gets from food; the body needs calories as "fuel" to perform all its functions.

Capsaicin An active component found in peppers and chillis.

Carbohydrate Starchy or sweet food, which provides the body with energy.

Cartilage A type of dense connective tissue that cushions

bones at the joints to absorb shock and prevent them from grating together.

Cholesterol A waxy substance found in red blood cells.

Choline A B-complex vitamin that is a constituent of lecithin; it is essential in the metabolism of fat, for good heart health and in the regulation of mood, appetite, behaviour and memory.

Chondroitin sulphate A complex molecule that gives cartilage the elastic, sponge-like quality that joints need to act as shock absorbers between bones.

Citric acid A plant acid that's an important component in the flavour of citrus fruit.

Cortisol A hormone produced by the adrenal glands, often called the "stress hormone".

Cruciferous A type of vegetable that's exceptionally rich in beneficial nutrients; includes cauliflower, Brussels sprouts and many dark green leafy vegetables.

Crustacean Seawater or freshwater creatures that have a hard outer shell and no backbone; includes lobsters, shrimps, crayfish and crabs.

Detoxification The body's natural process of eliminating toxic substances.

Dipeptides Muscle-building substances found in meat, especially turkey.

Diuretic Encourages the production of urine.

Docosahexaemoic acid (DHA) An omega-3 fatty acid found in fish.

Electrolyte A substance containing free ions, such as sodium, potassium, calcium and magnesium; commonly found in sports drinks that help to replenish the body's fluid levels.

Endurance The body's ability to exercise with minimal fatigue.

Enzyme A protein that facilitates the body's chemical reactions.

Essential amino acids Organic compounds that form the building blocks of protein and are vital to human health; the body can't produce them so they must be supplied by the diet.

Essential Fatty Acids (EFAs) Polyunsaturated fats the body can't manufacture, which are vital for healthy blood, skin, nerves and the functioning of the immune system.

Fat One of three food groups that we need to include in our diet; used for numerous purposes including cell maintenance and the absorption of certain vitamins.

Fibre Plant matter in food that the body does not absorb but that aids the process of digestion.

Flavonoids An umbrella term for the anti-inflammatory antioxidants found in many natural foods.

Folic acid Vitamin B9

Free radicals Highly reactive molecules that are damaging to the body and linked to causing degenerative diseases, such as cancer, as well as speeding up the ageing process.

Fructose A simple sugar found in honey and fruits.

Gingerol A source of spiciness in fresh root ginger.

Glucose The simplest form of sugar.

Glucosinolates Compounds found in vegetables in the cabbage family that have anti-cancer properties.

Gluten A protein found mainly in wheat, and in smaller amounts in barley and rye.

Glycaemic Index (GI) A system devised for ranking foods according to their effect on blood-sugar levels – foods with a high GI cause blood sugar to rise more quickly than medium- or low-GI foods.

Glycogen The form in which energy is stored in the muscles for later use.

Hesperin A cholesterol-lowering flavonoid with antioxidant and anti-inflammatory properties that is found in citrus fruit.

Homocysteine An amino acid used by the body in cellular metabolism and the manufacture of proteins; high levels of this substance have been found to be linked to an increased risk of heart disease and stroke.

Hormone A chemical substance released by the endocrine glands such as the thyroid and adrenal glands, and the ovaries, which travels through the bloodstream and affects the function of cells in other parts of the body.

Hull The dry outer covering of a fruit, seed or nut.

Hydrate To consume enough water to restore or maintain the body's fluid balance.

Insulin A hormone that regulates the body's blood-sugar levels.

Isoflavones Plant hormones that mimic the hormone oestrogen in the body.

Lactobacilli Friendly bacteria that live in the gut and support the immune system; bio-yogurt is a good source.

Lactose A natural sugar found in milk.

Lecithin A yellow phospholipid essential for the metabolism of fats; found in egg yolk and many plant and animal cells.

Leptin A hormone that plays a key role in regulating energy intake and expenditure; controls appetite and metabolism.

Lignans Antioxidant chemicals found in some plants, especially flaxseed; similar in structure to the hormone oestrogen, they mimic its actions in the body.

Lutein An antioxidant carotenoid important for eye health.

Lysine An essential amino acid found in proteins; important for growth, tissue repair, and the production of hormones, enzymes and antibodies.

Metabolism The process in the body that converts food into energy.

Mineral An inorganic chemical element, such as calcium, iron, potassium, sodium or zinc, required by the body for biochemical reactions; essential for optimal health.

Monounsaturated fat The healthiest type of fat found in food, which can help to lower cholesterol.

Niacin Vitamin B3

Nutrient A substance that can be metabolized in the body to provide energy and build tissue.

Oleic acid An omega-9 essential fatty acid, found in various animal and plant food sources, especially olives and olive oil.

Organic Food made according to strict production standards; crops are grown without the use of conventional pesticides or artificial fertilizers, free from human or industrial contamination and processed without ionizing radiation or food additives; animals are reared without antibiotics or growth hormones, and are fed healthily.

Osteoclasts The cells that break down bone.

Oxidation Exposure to oxygen that causes cell degeneration and decay.

Pantothenic acid Vitamin B5

Papain An enzyme found in papaya that aids the digestion of protein.

Pectin A type of soluble fibre in fruit and vegetables that lowers cholesterol levels.

Phospholipids Fats required for cell membranes and a healthy brain; found in eggs.

Phytoestrogen A plant compound that has similar, yet weaker, effects to those of the hormone oestrogen.

Phytonutrient A nutrient derived from a plant source.

Prebiotics Non-digestible fibres that are the energy source for the friendly bacteria in the colon.

Protein One of three food groups needed in our diet; essential for the growth and repair of muscle and tissue.

Pyridoxine Vitamin B6

Quercertin An anti-inflammatory flavonoid found in onions.

Rancid Having a rank taste and/or smell, commonly owing to the oxidation of oils or fats in food.

Resveratrol An antioxidant found in fruit and red wine, which has anti-cancer, anti-viral and anti-inflammatory properties.

Riboflavin Vitamin B2

Rutin A flavonoid antioxidant found in buckwheat, which helps to strengthen the blood vessels and fight heart disease.

Satiety The feeling of fullness or the disappearance of hunger after a meal.

Serotonin A chemical produced by nerve cells in the brain that lifts the mood; also found in some foods.

Thiamine Vitamin B1

Thyroid One of the largest endocrine glands in the body, found in the neck; it controls how quickly the body burns energy and makes proteins and how sensitive the body is to hormones.

Tryptophan An amino acid that the brain converts into the "feel-good" chemical, serotonin.

Vitamins Fat-soluble and water-soluble organic substances, such as beta-carotene, that are obtained naturally from plant and animal foods; essential in minute amounts for the normal growth and activity of the body.

Wholegrain Cereal grains that retain the bran and germ of the plant, such as wholemeal flour, brown rice and oatmeal.

index

Author's acknowledgments

Sarah would like to thank her husband, Anthony, and her three sons, Harry, Jonah and Luke, for their unfailing love and support during the writing of this book.

Publishers' acknowledgments

Thanks to The Fish Society (www.thefishsociety.co.uk) for providing crayfish and cod roe for the photo shoot.